Tan Men/Pale Women

Tan Men/Pale Women

COLOR AND GENDER IN ARCHAIC GREECE AND EGYPT, A COMPARATIVE APPROACH

Mary Ann Eaverly

THE UNIVERSITY OF MICHIGAN PRESS
ANN ARBOR

Published in the United States of America by
The University of Michigan Press
Manufactured in the United States of America
♾ Printed on acid-free paper

2017 2016 2015 2014 5 4 3 2

A CIP catalog record for this book is available from the British Library.

Library of Congress Cataloging-in-Publication Data

Eaverly, Mary Ann, 1957–
Tan men/pale women : color and gender in archaic Greece and Egypt, a comparative approach / Mary Ann Eaverly.
pages cm
Includes bibliographical references and index.
ISBN 978-0-472-11911-0 (hardback)
1. Gender identity in art. 2. Human skin color in art. 3. Polychromy—Egypt. 4. Vase-painting, Greek—Greece—Athens—Themes, motives. I. Title.
N8217.G397E28 2013
704.9'42093—dc23

2013025450

To Helen and Frank Eaverly: Aunt and Uncle Extraordinaire.
And to the Memory of Michael Eaverly

Acknowledgments

I did not know, in 1996, when a colleague asked me what I was working on, that in 2012 I would give the same answer: "color and gender in ancient painting." Thus, there are many people to thank. I greatly benefited from participation in the following conferences: *Fifth Gender in Archaeology Conference* (University of Wisconsin, Milwaukee), Oct. 9, 1998; *Sixth Gender in Archaeology Conference* (University of Northern Arizona Flagstaff), Oct. 24, 2000; *Colours in Antiquity Conference*, Department of Classics (University of Edinburgh), Sept. 10, 2001; *American Schools of Oriental Research Annual Meeting* (Boulder, Colorado), Nov. 16, 2001; *XVI International Congress of Classical Archaeology* (Harvard University), Aug. 25, 2003; *Gender and Diversity in Place/Feminism and Classics 4* (University of Arizona), May 28, 2004. I thank the conference organizers and my fellow participants.

I also thank John Younger for his invitation to speak as a panel member at the Third Annual Paul Rehak Symposium on Ancient Art (University of Kansas), Mar. 11, 2008. His comments and those of my fellow presenters, Mary Sturgeon and Janet Grossman, were very helpful.

I thank Ava Chitwood for her patient reading of drafts of my early thoughts on color and gender. Diana Boxer also critiqued early drafts. Beth Nakhai proved invaluable in helping me formulate my ideas about Egypt. Betty Banks delivered words of encouragement at exactly the right moment. Elizabeth McGowan provided valuable advice.

I also thank my past and present colleagues in the Classics Department at the University of Florida—Sheila Dickison, Karelisa Hartigan, Gareth Schmeling, Lewis Sussman, Judy Turner, David Young, Victoria Pagan (Chair), Eleni

Bozia, Tim Johnson, Kostas Kapparis, Nick Kontaridis, Jim Marks, Andrew Nichols, Jennifer Rea, Gonda Van Steen, Robert Wagman, and Andrew Wolpert, and also Barbara Barletta, Art History Department. They encouraged me and also provided a wonderful atmosphere in which to work. The Center for Women's Studies at the University of Florida, under the direction of Angel Kwolek-Folland, allowed me to garner valuable criticism through participation in their seminars. I also had many stimulating discussions with Marsha Bryant of the University of Florida English Department, with whom I co-authored a series of articles on the relationship between Classics, Egyptology, and Modernist poetry. I also thank the participants in my graduate Vase-Painting seminar for keeping me on my toes. In 2012, I was invited to be the Tracy Lecturer at the University of Illinois, Chicago Circle, and I thank Nanno Marinatios, Jennifer Tobin, and Karen Ros for the invitation and their helpful comments and questions. Going back to the dawn of my academic history I acknowledge John Pedley's stricture to his students to look at things with new eyes.

Dustin Heinen provided technical support as did Katherine Stone. I thank Erica Nikolaidis of Virgo Editorial for formatting. Annika Keller of Art Resource and Marta Fodor of The Boston Museum of Fine Arts provided invaluable help with illustrations. I also thank Ellen Bauerle and the staff and anonymous readers of the University of Michigan Press for their assistance.

Finally, and most importantly, there are two individuals without whom this book would never have been completed. I owe them a debt which I can never fully repay. Antoinette Emch-Deriaz gave generously and unstintingly of her expertise and time, patiently reading and critiquing every draft, always pushing me to greater clarity of thought and expression. My husband, Wayne Losano, provided loving support and technical writing and editing skills, standing by me despite my inability to master the nuances of comma use. I thank them both.

My research and travel were supported by a University of Florida Research Development Award and a University of Florida Humanities Enhancement Grant. The photographs were subsidized by a generous grant from the Rothman Family Foundation.

If I have left anyone out, it is inadvertent and only because of the passage of time. Any faults in this book are, of course, directly attributable to me.

Contents

List of Figures

Introduction

One stylistic feature is apparent to even the most casual observer of Athenian black-figure vase painting: the use of color to differentiate women from men. Male skin is the dark black color of the glaze, and female skin is painted with an added layer of white. Figure 1 is an example, but a quick walk through any museum gallery displaying black-figure vases confirms the ubiquity of this practice. While wall painting from this period is rare, some preserved panel paintings also show a darker skin tone for men than for women.[1] In addition, traces of dark paint for male figures appear among the poros pediments from the Acropolis.[2] Trained as a Classical archaeologist, I had been taught to look at the pale color of female flesh as a reflection of the secluded indoor lives of Athenian women as contrasted with the outdoor and thus "tanned" lives of men. The standard explanation offered in handbooks and classrooms was the one Martin Robertson presents in *A History of Greek Art*, a difference between "the sunburned frequenter of market-place and sports ground, field, sea and campaign; and the shadow-bred woman whose place is in the house."[3]

1. Painted panels: Metopes from Thermon, Temple of Apollo. National Museum Athens, J. Charbonneux. R. Martin and F. Villard, *Archaic Greek Art, 620–480 BC* (London: Thames and Hudson, 1971), Figs. 33–34. Corinthian plaque, Pitsa. National Museum Athens. Corinthian Plaque from Pitsa: National Museum Athens. *Archaic Greek Art*. Fig. 357. Clay plaque from the Athenian Acropolis, # 1037, J. Boardman, *Greek Art* (London: Thames and Hudson, 1985), Fig. 94.
2. See for example the Herakles from the Hydra pediment.
3. M. Robertson, *A History of Greek Art* (Cambridge: Cambridge University Press, 1975), 125. See also M. A. Eaverly, "The Iconography of Gender: Dark Men and Light Women in Archaic Painting," in *Common Ground: Archaeology, Art, Science and the Humanities, Proceedings of the XVII International Congress of Classical Archaeology*, ed. C. C. Mattusch, A. A. Donahue, and A. Brauer (Oxford: Oxford University Press, 2006), 23–26.

However, a look beyond Athens shows that male/female color differentiation is a widespread stylistic feature of ancient painting, one used throughout the art of the Mediterranean as well as in Egypt, where its use precedes its use in Archaic Greece. The question arises, then, whether the indoor/outdoor explanation holds true everywhere or even, in fact, in Greece. Just how "natural" is color-based gender differentiation? In fact, in a biological sense this distinction is very natural. Numerous studies of modern populations have revealed that women do in fact generally have lighter skin than men, regardless of the society in which they live, although what evolutionary role such dimorphism played is still hotly debated by anthropologists.[4] We might be dealing with a realistic depiction of human difference, and yet if we explore this phenomenon as depicted in art we see that in both Egypt and Greece this difference is emphasized such that women are not simply lighter than men, but are depicted in shades that are opposite to those used for men. In addition, in some periods in both of these ancient cultures, men and women are shown with the same skin color. This occurs in both areas in times during which the art is usually judged by modern scholars to be most naturalistic—the art of the Amarna period in Egypt and the red-figure vase painting from the Classical period in Greece.[5] This suggests that something beyond simple observation of nature is behind these depictions.

While Classical archaeologists have generally agreed that color differentiation represents a "natural" difference between men and women based on sun exposure, they are curiously silent about the disappearance of color differentiation in red-figure vase painting. This is especially surprising because the more realistic poses and details of musculature found in red figure are usually considered hallmarks of Greek naturalism. If vase painting at its most "naturalistic" abandons the concept of color differentiation, how natural can this convention be? According to *Webster's Dictionary*, the term *convention* in art refers to "accordance with an accepted manner, model or tradition."[6] But this begs the question of what makes a specific convention accepted, that is, what role does the convention fill that makes its use an acceptable standard for a society? To gain a clearer understanding of Archaic Greek society we need to interrogate the

4. For a summary see L. Madrigal and W. Kelly, "Human Skin-Color Sexual Dimorphism: A Test of the Sexual Selection Hypothesis," *American Journal of Physical Anthropology* 132 (2007): 470–82.

5. C. Cheal, an Egyptologist, notes the red-figure problem. C. Cheal, "The Meaning of Skin Color in Eighteenth Dynasty Egypt," in C. Fluehr-Lobban and K. Rhodes, eds., *Race and Identity in the Nile Valley* (Trenton: Red Sea Press, 2004), 59.

6. *Webster's New Universal Unabridged Dictionary* (New York: Barnes and Noble, 1996).

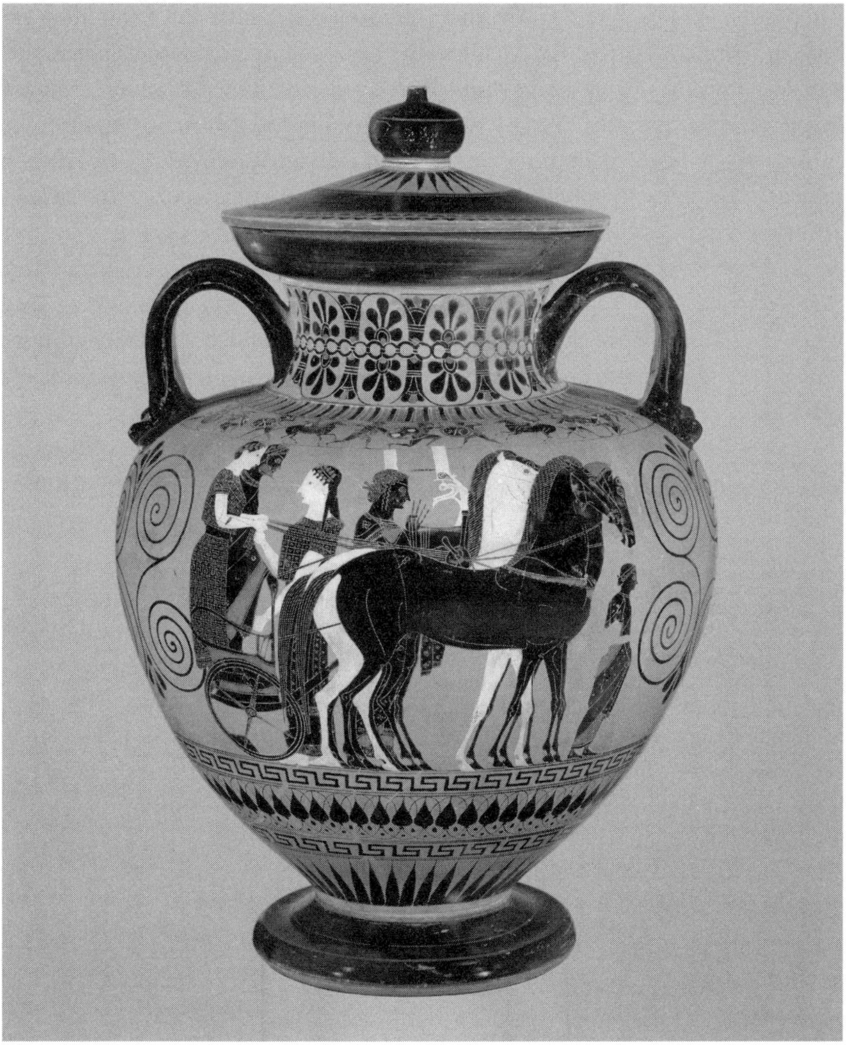

Fig. 1. Neck-amphora with lid: a man and a woman in a chariot are accompanied by a woman and kithara player. Exekias (6th BC) (attributed to). Greek, Attic, Archaic ca. 540 BC. Terracotta, h. 18 1/2 in (47 cm), diameter 9 3/4 in (24.8 cm). (Rogers Fund, 1917 (17.230.14a, b); Gift of J. D. Beazley, 1927 (27.16), 17.230.14a, b.) The Metropolitan Museum of Art, New York, NY, U.S.A. Image (© The Metropolitan Museum of Art/Art Resource, NY.)

vases more fully and not accept the simplest explanation. We know that art both mirrors and shapes underlying values. A standard practice such as male/female color differentiation may provide a distillation of these values if we are prepared to look closely. The key to understanding color differentiation lies in another observation by Martin Robertson. In *A History of Greek Art*, he further suggests that there may be more at work in this artistic practice than simple mimesis, that in fact color differentiation "is based on a difference of ideal and no doubt to some degree on actuality."[7] While the second part of the equation has been generally accepted, very little attention has been paid to the first part—the "difference of ideal." The question of the "ideal" behind the convention is the focus of this book. What world view does male/female color differentiation reflect?

The ubiquity of color/differentiation has kept scholars from questioning its meaning, and a thorough examination is long overdue. Simply because something is commonplace does not mean it need not be examined. It is precisely because male/female color differentiation was so widely used and accepted as necessary by ancient artists that it needs to be investigated more thoroughly. Something that a society takes as a commonplace should reflect basic ideas and beliefs held by that society. In attempting to ferret out these underlying beliefs, this book deals with a number of important questions: What relationship does male/female color differentiation have to the role of women in the ancient societies that used it? How does this artistic tool promote or reinforce ideas about the relative status of men and women? What ideology(ies) is (are) being expressed by the use of color differentiation? In what way did male/female color differentiation correspond to the reality of ancient Greek women's lives and the lives of women in other societies that used the convention? Why was it used so consistently throughout the Mediterranean over several millennia? What was its method of transmission? Was there an underlying need to define women as "other" in all the societies that used it and to do so in the same manner? Is color differentiation employed because all women in ancient Mediterranean societies were kept indoors?

The "naturalistic" indoor/outdoor explanation for gender-based color differentiation has precluded much investigation of what lay behind this artistic device. Accepting male/female color differentiation as a "realistic feature" suggests a reading of art as reality, a reading that is at best debatable. Can we actually consider these images to be realistic when other artistic features have been

---

7. M. Robertson, *A History of Greek Art*, 125.

shown to be at the very least stylized? For example, McNiven has shown that the limited repertoire of gestures used by figures on Archaic vases is gender-specific, reflecting underlying beliefs about the proper behavior for each sex.[8]

Pattern takes precedence over realistic detail in much of archaic art. Artistic depictions do not reflect actual appearance. An example in vase painting is the use of the profile eye (when a face is shown in profile, the entire eye is depicted). This stresses how important sight line and gaze were in the Archaic period.[9] Archaic sculpture also shows a reliance on pattern rather than realism. In early kouroi, kneecaps, ears, and hair are all more patterned than anatomically accurate. These statues are grounded in an ideology that exalts male beauty. Archaic Greek art uses patterns in a nuanced and symbolic manner. The ideal male figure is expressed not through conformation to reality but through an assemblage of beautifully patterned parts, which to the ancient Greeks made a perfect whole.

In the cultural milieu of Archaic Greece it is not to be expected that male/female color differentiation is simply a reflection of sun exposure. Rather it is an artistic choice made to illustrate an ideological belief system. This ideological underpinning has been largely ignored by scholars because we have been trained to look at Archaic art as a prelude to the more natural and highly admired art of the Classical period. Yet, as noted above, when Classical style appears in red-figure vase painting, male/female color differentiation is no longer used. If male/female color differentiation is not "natural," then what ideology does it support? As Pollock states, ideology "works by masking, naturalizing or flaunting a particular view of the world."[10] In the case of color differentiation, scholars have perhaps been seduced by the "naturalizing" (the sun exposure versus indoor living as the basis of color differentiation) without looking for the underlying viewpoint that made such a distinction seem "natural" in the first place. As Shelby Brown notes in "'Ways of Seeing' Women in Antiquity":

> Classical Archaeologists and ancient historians have too often examined stylistic and typological changes for their own sake, often on the basis of emotional

8. T. J. McNiven, "Behaving Like an Other: Telltale Gestures in Athenian Vase Painting," in *Not the Classical Ideal: Athens and the Construction of the Other in Greek Art*, ed. B. Cohen (Leiden: Brill Academic Publishers, 2000), 71–97.
9. On the gaze and sexuality, see E. D. Reeder, "Representing Women," in *Pandora: Women in Classical Greece*, ed. E. D. Reeder (Princeton: Princeton University Press, 1995), 125–26. On the importance of gaze in vase painting, see M. D. Stansbury-O'Donnell, *Vase Painting, Gender and Social Identity in Archaic Athens* (Cambridge: Cambridge University Press, 2006), 87.
10. S. Pollock, *Ancient Mesopotamia: The Eden that Never Was* (Cambridge: Cambridge University Press, 1999), 173.

and badly defined criteria. Many have assumed, at least as far as gender is concerned, that art simply reflects reality and so does not require much in the way of analysis or criticism.[11]

A reliance on art as reality certainly may explain why male/female color differentiation is usually accepted as an unexamined "given" of ancient art. The simple explanation (men go outside, women stay inside) has prevented any deeper investigation of what lay behind this artistic device. The underlying assumption behind the indoor/outdoor explanation is that ancient Athenian women were in fact secluded in the house. This flies counter to the many images showing women in a setting that is outside the house and to our knowledge of women's participation in religious festivals. Could male/female color differentiation mark an ideological seclusion of women rather than one strictly enforced in everyday life?

I began this book as a study of gender-based color differentiation in Archaic Greek painting. While the original focus of my study was Greece, I realized that I needed to expand the scope. Male/female color differentiation is not limited to Ancient Greek painting but is also found in Etruscan, Roman, and Egyptian painting. In a 1999 article[12] I suggested that the convention needed to be examined from a Pan-Mediterranean rather than from a purely Greek perspective. It had become clear to me that male/female color differentiation did not originate in Archaic Greece. Despite the assertion of Pliny the Elder that Eumaros, an otherwise unknown Athenian painter of the sixth century BC (N.H. 35.55–56),[13] was the first to distinguish between men and women by using color, the practice appears earlier in Egypt. By the Old Kingdom (3rd millennium BC), differentiating between male and female by color in freestanding and relief sculpture is standard practice in Egyptian art. Men are painted dark reddish brown, women a lighter color—either white or yellow. Egypt provides the opportunity to study male/female color differentiation as it develops during the early formative period of Egyptian history. In fact, as we shall see in Chapter 1, male/female color differentiation is one of the artistic features introduced to

---

11. S. Brown, "'Ways of Seeing' Women in Antiquity: An Introduction to Feminism in Classical Art and Archaeology," in *Naked Truths: Women, Sexuality and Gender in Classical Art and Archaeology*, ed. A. O. Koloski-Ostrow and C. L. Lyons (London: Routledge, 1997), 18.
12. M. A. Eaverly, "Color and Gender in Ancient Painting: A Pan-Mediterranean Approach," in *From the Ground Up: Beyond Gender Theory in Archaeology*, ed. N. Wicker and Bettina Arnold (Oxford: BAR S 812, 1999), 5–10.
13. J. Pollitt, *The Art of Ancient Greece: Sources and Documents* (Cambridge: Cambridge University Press, 1993), 125.

support the establishment of pharaonic rule. Egyptologists have long recognized the symbolic nature of color in Egyptian art where throughout millennia color is used to support underlying ideologies. Certain colors are, for example, associated with specific gods. Symbolic associations with the afterlife are particularly strong. Osiris, the god of the underworld, is often painted black, indicating the dark earth from which renewal comes. Turquoise was associated with the goddess Hathor and with the rising sun and was included in tombs as a symbol of the rebirth of the sun. While these aspects of color symbolism have been studied, Egyptian male/female color differentiation has not received as much attention.

Since Egyptian male/female color differentiation precedes Archaic Greek examples, it is only natural to ask if there is a connection between the two. Egyptian influence on early Greek art has long been recognized. But Near Eastern art also played a role. Although that region maintained close contacts with Egypt and was part of the Mediterranean koine, it does not consistently use color to differentiate between male and female. The fact that male/female color differentiation was not used by Near Eastern societies, which were in contact with the rest of the Mediterranean and could have adopted it, suggests that a strong ideological component rather than a natural component was involved. The picture, however, is by no means clear. Mesopotamia was not a single nation-state but rather was composed of city-states over which one ruler would briefly exert control. In contrast to Egypt, Mesopotamian art is not typically from a funerary context. Much is found in temples and also in the palaces of the rulers. Conclusions drawn from this region have to be tentative. Monumental painting is rare. While a substantial amount of sculpture is preserved from the region, bronze may have been the preferred material for monumental sculpture.[14] For stone sculpture, traces of paint are either poorly preserved or not recorded by excavators.

However, in the admittedly poorly preserved record of Near Eastern painting, male/female color differentiation is not consistently applied. In Near Eastern examples such as the investiture fresco of King Zimri-Lim from his palace at Mari, men and women are shown as dark brown in the main register, while in subsidiary registers some men are light and others dark. In Assyrian relief sculpture men are usually painted white.[15] Variation in color rather than a strictly binary division of male and female may also have an ideological basis.

14. A. Moortgat, *The Art of Ancient Mesopotamia* (London: Phaidon, 1969), 32.

15. Mari: A. Parrot, *Sumer* (London: Golden Press, 1960), Figs. 346–48. Assyria: A. Parrot, *Ninevah and Babylon* (London: Thames and Hudson, 1961), Figs. 344–47.

A study of Mesopotamian cylinder seals suggests that rather than a binary system emphasizing male and female as the primary categories, some cylinder seals show a figure identified by the authors as a third gender category.[16] If a binary gender system was not in place in the Near East, and color differentiation is linked to gender roles, one would expect that a two-color system of distinction between male and female might not be used in the Near East as it was in Greece and Egypt. Once Athenian vase painting adopts black-figure style there is little of the fluidity in skin color characteristic of Near Eastern wall painting, while such fluidity is exhibited by Proto-Corinthian and Corinthian vase painting.[17] In painting from Corinth, women are sometimes red and men often white. This suggests that while the appearance of dark male/light female color differentiation in Greece coincides with a period of influence from the Near East and Egypt, Egypt was more influential for Athenian vase painters.

This book therefore explores in particular the relationship between male/female color differentiation in Archaic Greece and Egypt. Egypt clearly has temporal priority. The earliest Egyptian examples predate the use of color differentiation in Archaic Greece. While attributing the Greek use of color differentiation to Egyptian influence may at first glance seem like a *post hoc, ergo propter hoc* argument, this book will show that a strong case can be made for Egyptian influence on Greek art in this instance. What is intriguing is whether the same meaning was attributed to the convention in both areas and in what ways, if any, it was changed in the Greek milieu. While Herodotus' well-known claim (2.35.1) that Egyptian laws and customs were the opposite of those in other parts of the world may be an exaggeration (he states that women did the marketing while men did the weaving and that women urinated standing while men did so squatting), it is clear from legal documents that Egyptian women had freedoms not available in the Mediterranean world.[18] They were, for ex-

16. S. Pollock and R. Bernbeck, "And They Said, Let Us Make Gods in Our Image: Gendered Ideologies in Ancient Mesopotamia," in *Reading the Body: Representations and Remains in the Archaeological Record*, ed. A. Rautman (Philadelphia: University of Pennsylvania Press, 2000), 150–64. On lack of binary concept for gender, see J. M. Asher-Greve, "The Essential Body: Mesopotamian Conceptions of the Gendered Body," in *Gender and the Body in the Ancient Mediterranean*, ed. M. Wyke (Oxford: Blackwell Publishers, 1998).

17. On such fluidity in Corinthian vase painting, see J. Boardman, *Early Greek Vase-Painting* (London: Thames and Hudson, 1988), 182, and J. Henderson, "Smashing Bodies: The Corinthian Tydeus and Ismene Amphora (Louvre E640)," in *Constructions of the Classical Body*, ed. J. I. Porter (Ann Arbor: University of Michigan Press, 1999), 19–49.

18. On the legal status of Egyptian women, see J. Johnston, "The Legal Status of Women in Ancient Egypt," in *Mistress of the House, Mistress of Heaven: Women in Ancient Egypt*, ed. A. K. Capel and G. E. Markoe (New York: Hudson Hill Press, 1996), 175–86.

ample, independent legal persons who, unlike Greek women, did not need a male guardian. They were also free to own property in their own right. Yet both ancient societies deemed it important to differentiate between men and women by the color convention.

Egypt also provides a clear link between male/female color differentiation and ideology. This link first appears when pharaonic ideology is being created, which emphasizes the joining of opposites for the creation of a harmonic universe with pharaoh as its guarantor. Male and female are painted in colors that are considered opposites. The union of these opposites promotes the continuation and order of the universe. In Egypt the use of male/female color differentiation is clearly linked to ideology, and it changes when the ideology changes. Two periods that illustrate this most clearly are the reigns of Hatshepsut and of Akhenaten. As we shall see in Chapter 2, Hatshepsut (Eighteenth Dynasty) adjusts the male/female color convention to support her attempts at legitimizing her exceptional reign. She is a female holding an office traditionally gendered male. The coloring of her images is an important part of promoting her message. Are her images painted the traditional female colors (yellow and white) or the color (dark reddish brown) associated with males and thus the "correct" color for the holder of the office of pharaoh? A second key period in Egyptian art, which I discuss in Chapter 2, is the reign of the pharaoh Akhenaten, a period in which the religious system of the Egyptians was radically reorganized—thus causing a clear shift in ideology. What is the significance of the abandonment of the use of male/female color differentiation during this period?

My comparative approach between Greek and Egyptian monuments is not new. The relationship between Greek and Egyptian art has been the subject of many studies that have shown the connection between Egypt and Greece's adoption of monumental stone architecture and sculpture during the Orientalizing period.[19] The limits of the evidence produce numerous problems. Almost no monumental painting survives from Greece in this period, and we must rely on vase painting and some hints of color from sculpture. This is in marked contrast to the huge corpus of wall painting, painted relief, and painted freestanding sculpture preserved in Egypt. In addition, vase painting was not part of the Egyptian artistic repertoire during the period in question. One risks being faulted for comparing items that at first glance might not seem comparable.

19. For connections between Greece and Egypt, see J. M. Hurwit, *The Art and Culture of Early Greece, 1100–480 B.C.* (Ithaca: Cornell University Press, 1985), 192–97. See also B. S. Ridgway, *The Archaic Style in Greek Sculpture* (Chicago: Ares Publications, 1975), 29–34.

However, the fact that color differentiation crosses media lines indicates its importance. The exact nature of the relationship between Egypt and Greece has also been the subject of some controversy, as in Martin Bernal's *Black Athena*,[20] which attributes almost all of the philosophical, artistic, and religious elements that most scholars consider uniquely Greek to Egyptian conquest and colonization. (I acknowledge Greece's clear debt to Egypt but don't follow Bernal's model. My model is one of influence rather than conquest.)

Specific studies of the relationship between Greece and Egypt have also been conducted for painting. One can look at Schäfer's early study of the principles of Egyptian art to see the comparative method.[21] However, Schäfer's study focuses primarily on Egypt's failure to develop techniques of perspective and illusionism so characteristic of the "Greek Revolution," that is, the shift to mimesis in Classical Greek art. Greek "advances" are also the focus of subsequent comparative work on Egyptian and Greek painting (see, for example, E. H. Gombrich's fundamental study of iconology, *Art and Illusion*). Here Egyptian painting—lacking the development of perspective and shadow exhibited by Greek painting, or at least in descriptions of the Greek paintings in Roman authors such as Pliny—is found wanting. The emphasis on what Gombrich calls the "uniqueness of Greek art" in this respect has tended to overshadow all other features. Because of this overriding interest in the development of Greek painting, Gombrich does not pursue his own cogent observation regarding the Egyptian use of color to differentiate gender: "The real flesh tone of the person portrayed obviously mattered as little in this context as the real colour of a river matters to the cartographer."[22] He is not interested in the underlying meaning behind the Egyptian practice of color differentiation.

In fact, the Egyptian creation of a symbolic system of representation has generally been given short shrift by Classical scholars who are usually more focused on the development of illusionistic techniques in Greek painting. Some scholars, such as Nelson Goodman,[23] have taken exception to the valuation of Western (Greco-Roman based) painting as more realistic than other systems of painting, but "naturalism" and "realism" in Greek painting (and sculpture) are a continued emphasis in Classical scholarship. As a result, color differentia-

20. M. Bernal, *Black Athena: The Afro-Asiatic Roots of Classical Civilization* (New Brunswick: Rutgers, 1987).
21. H. Schäfer, *Principles of Egyptian Art*, ed. J. Baines (Oxford: Griffith Institute, 1974).
22. E. H. Gombrich, *Art and Illusion* (Baltimore: Johns Hopkins University Press, 1977), 103.
23. N. Goodman, *Languages of Art* (Indianapolis: Hackett Publishing, 1976).

tion—a feature shared by Egypt, with its symbolically based art, and Archaic Greece, whose art is perceived as a step on the road to naturalism—has been overlooked. What does this shared artistic practice of color differentiation say about the connection between the two areas? What type of influence or cross-cultural transmission was at work?

The differing circumstances of production of Egyptian and Greek painting must also be considered. The Egyptian material primarily comes from tombs and was part of the funerary equipment and decoration designed to ensure the afterlife of the deceased. While many Athenian vases were found in tombs, they were not specifically produced for use as grave goods. Instead, they were used for storage, drinking, and other quotidian functions. However, the fact that the male/female color differentiation was used in differing circumstances in these two ancient societies makes an examination of its meaning even more significant.

The influence and transmission of ideas is another slippery scholarly area that this book will consider. Martin Bernal's *Black Athena* supports a conquest/colonization role for Egypt in relationship to Greece, which I, along with most Classical archaeologists, reject. Sarah Morris emphasizes that a linguistic model, namely *calque*, a loan followed by translation into a native idiom, more aptly describes the situation.[24] An examination of the color convention is an important contribution to the discussion of how one civilization "influences" another.

The reader may have noticed that I have yet made no mention of Bronze Age Greek examples of the color convention. While I will not totally ignore the Bronze Age in this study, it will serve only a subsidiary role. Bronze Age material presents problems that are beyond the scope of this book. Without substantial written sources, it is even more difficult to evaluate gender roles for this period than it is for Archaic Greece. The question of just how much, if any, the Bronze Age influenced Greece across the Dark Ages remains a point of scholarly controversy. The range of theories concerning the relationship between the two periods includes seeing them as part of a broad continuum, admitting some intermittent influence of Bronze Age remains, and accepting a total break between Bronze Age and Dark Age civilization.[25] Langdon's study of Dark Age

24. S. Morris, *Daidalos and the Origins of Greek Art* (Princeton: Princeton University Press, 1992), 98.

25. Continuum: S. Morris, *Daidalos and the Origins of Greek Art*, 109. Intermittent: J. Boardman, *The Greeks Overseas* (London: Thames and Hudson, 1980), 14. Break: I. Morris, *Archaeology as Cultural History: Words and Things in Iron Age Greece* (Malden, MA: Wiley-Blackwell, 2000), 207.

iconography in Geometric vase painting, *Art and Identity in Dark Age Greece, 1100–700 B.C.E.*, suggests that Bronze Age motifs are not common. Instead, Geometric art works out a new idiom of expression befitting the massive changes in societal order that took place during that period. Geometric vase painting does not depict figures in the same way as Bronze Age painting. Human figures are rendered as Geometric forms. Male and female are differentiated by costume and gesture, but not by color. It is only when contact with Egypt occurs during the subsequent Orientalizing period that male/female color differentiation reappears in the artistic repertoire. I see Archaic art as expressing the social tensions of its own age, in particular stresses in the roles of male and female through the artistic devices such as male/female color differentiation displayed in black-figure vase painting. It is not a throwback to Bronze Age painting but rather a re-interpretation of a stylistic device long used in Egypt. Here again questions need to be answered. Why did the Greeks consider this Egyptian practice something worth adopting at this time? What underlying societal needs did it fill? Does this use of color indicate a belief in a fundamental difference between men and women? To answer these questions I need to focus on literary as well as artistic evidence to understand the roles of women in Archaic Athenian society.

Literary sources pose many difficulties since many of our literary sources are Classical rather than Archaic. Eleanor Irwin's pioneering study *Colour Terms in Greek Poetry* (1974) provides a source for understanding color in Athenian society. She shows the various uses poets made of the Greek color vocabulary, in particular the strong contrast between light and dark in descriptions of women and men. That this contrast was particularly important in Athens is suggested by the above-mentioned attribution by Pliny the Elder of the invention of male/female color differentiation to a sixth-century BC *Athenian* painter named Eumaros.[26] While his chronology is wrong, Pliny the Elder's choice of locale may reflect an understanding of the sharp division between male and female roles in Athenian society. As noted above, male/female color differentiation disappears in red figure, which is the "cutting edge" style for vase painting in the Classical period. Medical and philosophical texts, again later than the Archaic period, discuss fundamental differences between male and female that are given a basis in physiology and temperament. Men and women were con-

26. E. Sellers, *The Elder Pliny's Chapters on the History of Art*, translated by K. Jex-Blake (New York: Macmillan, 1976), xxviii–xxix. J. Pollitt, *The Art of Ancient Greece: Sources and Documents* (Cambridge: Cambridge University Press, 1993), 125.

sidered to be temperamentally different because of different body compositions.[27] Were these ideas current during the Archaic period? Does male/female color differentiation refer to biological ideas or societal beliefs? Is it, as in Egypt, part of a religious view of the cosmos?

Much important work has been done on the presentation of women in ancient art and on approaches to the study of gender in archaeology. Feminist Classical scholars, beginning with Sarah Pomeroy's *Goddesses, Wives, Whores and Slaves: Women in Classical Antiquity* (1975), have sought first to call attention to women in the ancient record and then to formulate ways to understand methods of gender construction and representation. Many of these studies are based on the radical shift in thinking that occurred in response to John Berger's *Ways of Seeing* (1972), which helped to formulate the question of the "male gaze" as a determinative influence on the choice of artistic subjects and their presentation.[28] Identifying the significance of the viewer of art opened the door to feminist art historians' exploration of the power dynamic involved in the choice of artistic subject and in the way subjects are viewed. Among many works I mention only a few: *Women in the Classical World: Image and Text*, Elaine Fathom et al. (1994); *Sexuality in Ancient Art*, edited by N. B. Kampen; and *Naked Truths: Women, Sexuality and Gender in Classical Art*, edited by A. O. Koloski-Ostrow. Specific vase-painting studies have also discussed the types of scenes in which women appear on Greek vases and the relationship of the types of scenes depicted to what we know of ancient Greek women's actual lives (see, for example, Gloria Pinney's *Figures of Speech, Men and Maidens in Ancient Greece* and Sian Lewis's *The Athenian Woman: An Iconographic Handbook*. In addition, Egyptologists have conducted important studies of women's roles in ancient Egypt. Examples include *Women in Ancient Egypt*, by G. Robins; *Mistress of the House, Mistress of Heaven: Women in Ancient Egypt*, edited by A. Capel and G. Markoe; and *Silent Images: Women in Pharaonic Egypt* (New York, 2000) by Z. Hawass.[29]

Feminist Egyptologists, Classicists, and anthropologists have taken the lead

27. On Classical views on women's physiology, see L. D. Jones, "The Classical Construct of the Female Body in Classical Greek Science," in *Women's History and Ancient History*, ed. S. B. Pomeroy (Chapel Hill: University of North Carolina Press, 1991), 110–37.

28. On this point see S. Brown, "Women in Antiquity: An Introduction to Feminism in Classical Art and Archaeology," in *Naked Truths: Women, Sexuality and Gender in Classical Art and Archaeology*, ed. A. O. Koloski-Ostrow and C. L. Lyons (London: Routledge, 1997), 14–18.

29. See also G. Robins, "Gender Roles," in D. Redford, ed., *The Oxford Encyclopedia of Ancient Egypt*, Vol. 2 (Oxford: Oxford University Press, 2000), 12–16, and L. Manniche, "Sexuality," in Redford, *The Oxford Encyclopedia of Ancient Egypt*, Vol. 3 (Oxford: Oxford University Press, 2000), 274–77.

in examining gender construction across cultures. See, for example, *Engendering Archaeology, Women and Prehistory* (1991); *Gender in Archaeology* (1997); and *From the Ground Up: Beyond Gender Theory in Archaeology* (1999). Sue Langdon has emphasized the importance of gender roles in the creation of Greek Geometric art.[30] However, the use of the color convention in the construction of gender roles has not been addressed in any of these important studies.

Color in ancient painting has also become a hot topic in recent years. A major contribution to the discussion is *Color and Culture* by J. Gage (1993), which, although it discusses color in Greek painting and, provides a survey from antiquity through modern Abstract art does not discuss Egypt. Several conferences (cf. *Colour and Painting in Ancient Egypt*, British Museum, 1996; *Colour in the Ancient Mediterranean World*, Edinburgh, 2001; *Colour in Ancient Greece*, Thessaloniki, 2002) have been held to address color use and symbolism in the ancient world, but again little mention has been made of the color convention.[31] Polychromy in early Greek sculpture has also received scholarly attention (see, for example, V. Manzelli, *La Policromia nella Statuaria Greca Arcaica*, Rome, 1994). However, preservation has made the task of identifying original color schemes in sculpture very difficult. Precipitated by ever-more-sophisticated scientific analysis, in particular the work of Vincenz Brinkmann, which has revealed traces of pigment on sculpture and architecture that had been lost to the unaided eye, recent scholarship has seen an explosion of studies of the use of color in Greek sculpture. While previous generations of scholars concentrated on literary accounts by Roman writers, such as Pliny, to try to visualize lost Greek wall paintings, new excavations have uncovered examples of Greek wall painting, especially in Macedonia. Vase-painting scholars have turned to studying the specialized techniques that added polychromy to black- and red-figure vases.[32] Yet this most common phenomenon—dark men and light women—has been almost completely overlooked.

---

30. S. Langdon, *Art and Identity in Dark Age Greece, 1100–700 B.C.E.* (Cambridge: Cambridge University Press, 2008).
31. Publications: W. V. Davies, ed., *Colour and Painting in Ancient Egypt* (London: British Museum Press, 2001); M. A. Tiverios and D. S. Tsiafakis, eds., *Color in Ancient Greece* (Thessaloniki, 2002); and L. Cleland and K. Stears, eds., *Colour in the Ancient Mediterranean World*, BAR International Series 1267 (Oxford: British Archaeological Reports, 2004).
32. B. Cohen, ed., *The Colors of Clay: Special Techniques in Athenian Vases* (Los Angeles: Getty Museum, 2006).

There have also been significant anthropological and linguistic studies of color terminology. Berlin and Kay examined the relationship between the human ability to see colors versus the terms that are actually used in any given language to name those colors. Their work showed that while languages are generally limited to from two to eleven color terms, human beings are able to perceive thousands more colors.[33] The labeling of color is thus a cultural construct. Scholars such as Baines[34] and Wilkinson[35] have worked specifically with the meanings and use of color terms in Egypt, revealing a rich symbolic use of color although not focusing specifically on color and gender.

All of these studies provide a valuable resource for my study of male/female color differentiation. Recent studies of domestic architecture also shed light on the question of the seclusion of Athenian women. Archaeologists have reexamined the picture of separate men's and women's quarters in Athenian houses. All of these studies provide a firm background against which to examine color differentiation and—predicated on my belief that something more than sun exposure is at the root of color as gender indicator—make this the ideal time to conduct such a study.

This book has further significance for another important topic: race. Earlier generations of scholars sought to identify Egyptians racially based on the skin color depicted in their paintings.[36] For example, in a 1941 *National Geographic Magazine* article on daily life in ancient Egypt, the illustrations deliberately lightened the skin of male Egyptians in reproductions of wall paintings to ensure that viewers saw Egyptian civilization as white.[37] Egyptian skin color continues to be a controversial topic. In 2007 protestors picketed an exhibition of Tutankhamun at the Franklin Institute in Philadelphia on the grounds that the light-skinned model of the pharaoh presented by the museum was racist because it did not show his true African ethnicity (*Philadelphia Daily News*, May

33. B. Berlin and P. Kay, *Basic Color Terms: Their Universality and Evolution* (Berkeley: CSLI, 1969). See also C. L. Hardin and L. Maffi, eds., *Color Categories in Thought and Language* (Cambridge: Cambridge University Press, 1997).

34. J. Baines, "Color Terminology and Color Classification: Ancient Egyptian Color Terminology and Polychromy," *American Anthropologist* 87 (1985): 282–97; J. Baines, *Visual and Written Culture in Ancient Egypt* (New York: Oxford University Press, 2007).

35. R. H. Wilkinson, *Symbol and Magic in Egyptian Art* (London: Thames and Hudson, 1994).

36. For newer thinking see C. Cheal, "The Meaning of Skin Color in Eighteenth Dynasty Egypt," in *Race and Identity in the Nile Valley*, ed. C. Fluehr-Lobban and K. Rhodes (Trenton: Red Sea Press, 2004), 50–57.

37. B. Trigger, "Egyptology, Ancient Egypt and the American Imagination," in *The American Discovery of Ancient Egypt*, ed. N. Thomas (Los Angeles: Los Angeles County Museum, 1995), 32.

21, 2007, Stephanie Farr). While the concept of race is disappearing as a category in anthropological studies, it is still important to understand that if color is used in a symbolic manner it should not be taken as a racial marker.

This examination of the use of male/female color differentiation from its origin in Egypt through its use in Archaic Greece is my attempt to answer the questions posed above. Questions of underlying meaning, ideology, gender construction, and cross-cultural transmission are big questions, and I may be faulted for taking on such a broad topic, especially since I am neither an Egyptologist nor a vase-painting specialist. However, in this age of archaeological specialization, sometimes the big picture is, to our detriment I think, lost. As Shelby Brown notes:

> Ultimately, classical archaeology's success at "engendering" the field will very largely depend upon an increased willingness to communicate internally and to break down arbitrary barriers between disciplines. Only then will we be able to make meaningful choices from among the many "ways of seeing" women in antiquity.[38]

In my previous book (*Archaic Greek Equestrian Sculpture*, Ann Arbor, 1996) I focused on the twenty-some pieces of extant early equestrian sculpture to try to unravel possible identities and symbolism of that type of sculpture and connected them specifically to the aristocratic milieu of Athens. Although I worked with fewer objects, I was looking at the same kind of problems, the big questions of the construction of meaning through art.

Because this book marks another attempt on my part to deal with large issues it may fall short on some of the details. I cannot examine every example of Egyptian painting or every Greek vase. However, I hope that raising these questions and in some cases answering them will provide an important tool for understanding gender roles in Ancient Greece and Egypt and the transmission of ideas from one society to another.

The first two chapters focus on Egypt. Chapter 1, "Establishing the Norm—Old Kingdom Precedents," discusses the beginning of the color convention in Egypt, its full development in the Old Kingdom, and its relationship to the status of women. Chapter 2, "The Exception That Proves the Rule—Hatshepsut

38. S. Brown, "Women in Antiquity: An Introduction to Feminism in Classical Art and Archaeology," in *Naked Truths: Women, Sexuality and Gender in Classical Art and Archaeology*, ed. A. O. Koloski-Ostrow and C. L. Lyons (London: Routledge, 1997), 26.

and Akhenaten," examines two "crisis" points in the use of the convention—the rule of the female pharaoh Hatshepsut (i.e., What happens to the convention when the occupant of a position traditionally gendered male is a woman?) and the rule of the "heretic" pharaoh Akhenaten (What happens to the color convention when the religious foundation of Egyptian society is altered?).

The second part focuses on Archaic Greece. Chapter 3, "Establishing the Norm—the Road to Attic Black Figure," explores the beginning of the color convention in Greece, the role of Egyptian influence during the Orientalizing period, and the use of the convention in Athenian black figure in relationship to the status of women. Chapter 4, "The Exception That Proves the Rule—Attic Red Figure," discusses the abandonment of the convention in red figure and its significance. The Conclusion addresses the significance of the use of color as gender indicator in these two ancient societies and points to further questions. Greece and Egypt are not the only ancient societies that use this artistic feature. Further work remains to be done to understand male/female color differentiation's prevalence in Etruscan and Roman painting (both heavily influenced by Greek art) and to understand why this distinction even appears in sixteenth-century European painting.[39] To fully understand color as a persistent signifier of fundamental difference between male and female, I start at the beginning with the Egyptians.

A Note on the Illustrations

In a world of unlimited resources this book would have been lavishly illustrated with color images. It is not, but I hope that the limited number of black and white photos do help the reader understand the dark/light male/female color contrast that is the book's focus. The bibliography contains sources for examining the works cited in color.

39. Z. Filipzak, in *Hot Dry Men, Cold Wet Women: The Theory of Humors in Western European Art, 1575–1700* (New York: American Federation of Arts, 1997), connects male/female color differentiation in seventeenth-century European painting to Galen and ancient medical ideas, but does not explore earlier uses of Egyptian or Greek color differentiation.

CHAPTER 1

Egypt

Establishing the Norm—Old Kingdom Precedents

Most handbooks of ancient Greek art list Egypt as the inspiration for the use of male/female color differentiation in Archaic Greek painting. An Egyptian source has been a consistent observation as early as Mary Hamilton Swindler's *Ancient Painting*, written in 1929. She observes that "among the earliest Greek paintings . . . sexes were early distinguished by color. . . . This practice was probably derived from Egypt."[1] The practice to which Swindler refers is the use of dark-reddish paint for male flesh and a lighter color—either yellow or white—for female flesh, as seen in Figure 2. More than fifty years after Swindler, John Boardman followed the same path, noting in *Athenian Black Figure Vases*, "The male=red, female=white conventions of Egyptian art may have had some direct effect here,"[2] that is, in Greek painting. Yet while Egypt is generally indicated as the source for male/female color differentiation, little attention has been paid to what role this artistic choice played in Egyptian art, let alone why the Greeks might have considered it something worth borrowing.[3] Why did the Egyptians need an additional layer of differentiation between male and female beyond costume or secondary sexual characteristics? What world view did such a distinction between male and female support?

These questions presuppose that the use of color to differentiate between men and women was not arbitrary but was instead a deliberate choice that reflected Egyptian views about the relationship between male and female. The use

1. M. H. Swindler, *Ancient Painting* (New Haven: AMS Press, 1929), 135–36.
2. J. Boardman, *Athenian Black Figure Vases* (London: Thames and Hudson, 1974), 16.
3. A notable exception is C. Cheal, "The Meaning of Skin Color in Eighteenth Dynasty Egypt," in *Race and Identity in the Nile Valley*, ed. C. Fluehr-Lobban and K. Rhodes (Trenton: Red Sea Press, 2004), 47–70.

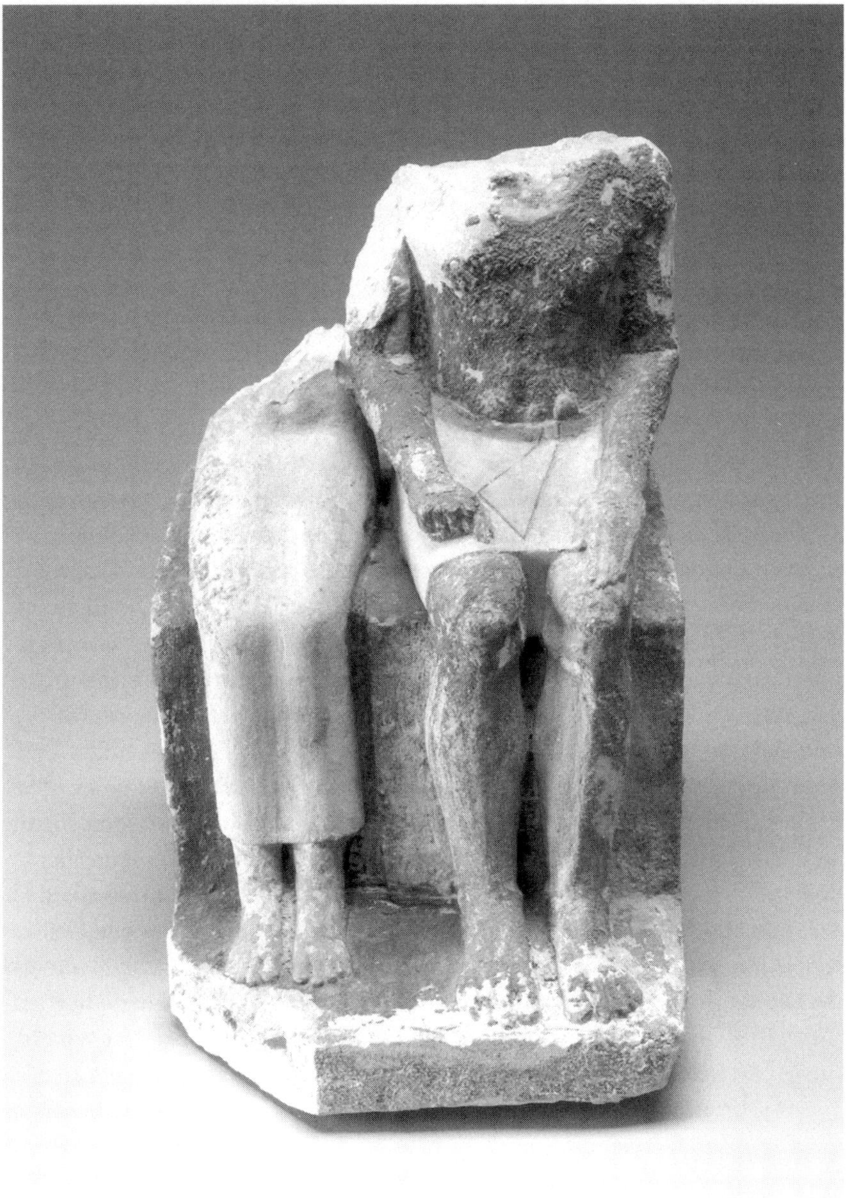

Fig. 2. Seated pair statue of man and wife. Egyptian, Old Kingdom, Fifth Dynasty, 2465–2150 BC. Find-spot: Egypt, Giza, Tomb G 2231/X. Limestone. Height × width × depth: 9 1/16 × 5 5/16 × 6 5/16 in (23 × 13.5 × 16 cm). (Museum of Fine Arts, Boston Harvard University—Boston Museum of Fine Arts Expedition, 12.1485.)

of artistic images to promote ideology is not a radical concept in the study of Egyptian art. Male/female color differentiation is just one of many representational formulae used in Egyptian painting and sculpture. Aspects of figures, such as scale and relative position, are manipulated to express status. Size is equivalent to importance. In any scene the taller figures have higher status. In battle scenes a giant pharaoh smites enemies who are often shown in miniature. Tomb owners are much larger than the servant figures shown performing tasks for them.[4]

Such a difference in scale is an obvious expression of dominant power in a relationship, but there are also more subtle ways of indicating the status of figures in painting and relief. As Robins has shown, important figures (e.g., the owner of a tomb as opposed to his servants) generally face right in relief sculpture and paintings. This directional orientation may be a reflection of the fact that hieroglyphic writing is also oriented to the right.[5] In Egypt, writing and sculpture are closely connected. Most decorated monuments combine sculpture and hieroglyphs. Hieroglyphic inscriptions are also carved on freestanding statues. Tomb statues are provided with the name and title of the person represented. The combination of writing and sculpture enhances the meaning of the statue. The carved name allows the gods to recognize the individual depicted just as does the portrait-like quality of the sculptural likeness. Together, sculpture and hieroglyphs create a symbolic language.

Hieroglyphs also reveal the multivalent and nuanced nature of Egyptian images. A hieroglyphic sign is not always read as the image depicted. Of the approximately 600 pictograms used, some function as words and others carry only phonetic meaning.In the Egyptian language a character can thus stand for the thing it represents or for a sound.[6] The Egyptian world view is thus attuned to a subtle interplay between image and idea through writing and sculptural depictions. Although the signs of hieroglyphic script are in fact miniature pictures, they do not always function in a one-to-one correlation of word with image. An image of a bird does not necessarily represent the word for bird. In

4. Examples: Pharaoh smiting: King Thutmose III, relief, 7th pylon of temple of Amun at Karnak, Eighteenth Dynasty ca. 1450 BC, J. Malek, *Egypt: 4000 Years of Art* (London: Phaidon Press, 2003), Figs. 142–43. Tomb owner: Tomb of Nebamun (T90) Nebamun oversees cattle workers, C. K. Wilkinson and M. Hill, *Egyptian Wall Paintings* (New York: Abbeville Press, 1983), Fig. 28.

5. G. Robins, "Some Principles of Compositional Dominance and Gender Hierarchy in Egyptian Art," *Journal of the American Research Center in Egypt 31* (1994): 33.

6. On the relationship between writing and art, see J. Baines, *Visual and Written Culture in Ancient Egypt* (New York: Oxford University Press, 2007), especially p. 198.

fact a depiction of an animal might stand for the god with which that particular animal is associated. Each hieroglyph can also function as a phoneme for a specific sound that makes up another word or as a determinative added to a group of signs to modify meaning. For example, the addition of walking legs indicated that a word signified motion. The symbol of a clenched hand can stand for "fist" but also for ideas associated with a fist such as grasping or seizing.[7] This combination of picture, sound, and metaphor (an image of an object used to suggest another object) indicates a world view in which images cannot be "read" simply on the basis of their appearance.[8]

This linguistic phenomenon surely carried over to artistic depictions. An image has a significance beyond its surface appearance. We have already seen how height and other features such as relative position of figures are manipulated in sculpture to show the power relationship between different individuals. Such images cannot be interpreted as simply descriptions of actual height difference, but instead the viewer has to apply an additional layer of meaning, in the same way that hieroglyphic writing presupposes a more sophisticated interpretation than simply equating a hieroglyphic character with the image it represents.

Like sculpture, hieroglyphs help to promote standardized depictions through their connection to the underlying conceptual frameworks of ancient Egyptian society. They provide a visual as well as a linguistic representation of the way in which the Egyptians categorized the world. As Frandsen notes, "Categorization is a matter of paramount importance. People cannot think about the world, let alone act within it, unless they divide it into classes."[9] With hieroglyphs, color also plays a role. The meaning of the pictograms is carried not only by the image itself but also by the paint that decorates the individual characters. All of the signs are painted. The pictorial nature of hieroglyphic writing helped to create such a symbolic color vocabulary. As Wilkinson observes:

> The dual usage of colors—on the one hand where objects are given the same hue as they appear in nature, and on the other, where objects are assigned colors to which they are symbolically linked—is clearly found in the colors used in the

7. R. H. Wilkinson, *Symbol and Magic in Egyptian Art* (London: Thames and Hudson, 1994), 155–57, and R. H. Wilkinson, *Reading Egyptian Art* (London: Thames and Hudson, 1982), 55.
8. P. J. Frandsen, "On Categorization and Metaphorical Structuring: Some Remarks on Egyptian Art and Language," *Cambridge Archaeological Journal* 7, No. 1: (1977): 71–10; see especially p. 81 on the role of metaphor.
9. Ibid., 81.

depiction of Egyptian hieroglyphs. Each hieroglyph—itself a miniature picture—in the Egyptians' written language had its own color combination which was faithfully kept whenever multiple colors were used in formal inscriptions or in decorative elements.[10]

However, hieroglyphic coloring also indicates subsidiary status for women. Male dark-brown coloring is the "default setting" for hieroglyphs that indicate parts of the human body. For example, the sign for *arm* is an extended arm painted dark reddish-brown, even if the text itself refers to a woman's arm. One can see an analogous practice in the English language. Until fairly recently, the term *mankind* or *man* was used to refer to humanity in general. For example, in the 1960s television show *Star Trek*, the male *and* female crew of the starship Enterprise "boldly go where no *man* has gone before." However, in the 2009 *Star Trek* film, societal changes in the status of women are reflected in the fact that the same crew now goes "where *no one* has gone before." In hieroglyphic inscriptions accompanying statues or reliefs, a man's offices are stressed by listing his titles, while for women the relationship to the husband is stressed.[11]

In art, hierarchical depictions also help to differentiate between male and female. Men are depicted in action poses, striding, while women stand with feet close together. In relief sculpture Robins points to "a notion of gender hierarchy that is often expressed by means of compositional dominance."[12] As she points out, in statuary groups the figures on the right are the more powerful figures and are usually male. For example, Pharaoh is almost always on the right. If a couple is shown overlapping, the forward position is the dominant one and usually occupied by the man, as in Figure 3.

Not all of these compositional devices remain static throughout Egyptian history. Changes may suggest a link to changes in ideology. In Early Old Kingdom seated statue groups consisting of pairs of men and women (usually husband and wife, but also sometimes mother and son as in Figure 4), there is no height dichotomy between men and women. Here isocephaly is an organizing principle: husband and wife are shown as the same height. This cannot be read as an attempt at "naturalism" since on average in human populations men tend to be taller than women. This use of isocephaly as an artistic device is particu-

10. R. H. Wilkinson, *Symbol and Magic in Egyptian Art*, 110.

11. G. Robins, "Some Principles of Compositional Dominance and Gender Hierarchy in Egyptian Art," *Journal of the American Research Center in Egypt*, 31 (1994): 33.

12. Ibid., 33.

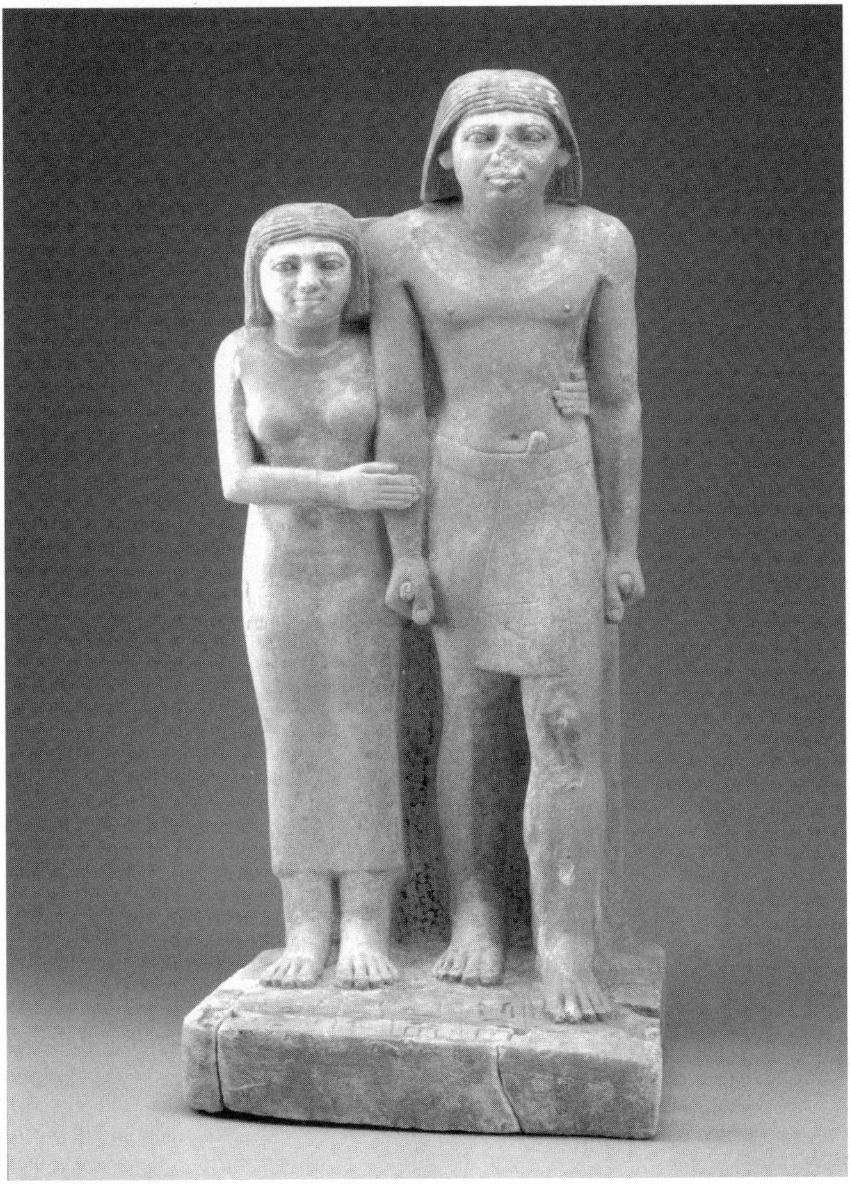

Fig. 3. Pair statue of Nefu and Khenetemsetju. Egyptian, Old Kingdom, Fifth Dynasty, reign of Niussera to Una, 2455–2350 BC. Find-spot: Egypt, Giza, Tomb G 7946. Limestone. Height × width × depth: 29 x 13 1/8 × 11 15/16 in (73.6 × 33.3 × 30.4 cm). (Museum of Fine Arts, Boston, Harvard University—Boston Museum of Fine Arts Expedition, 31.777.)

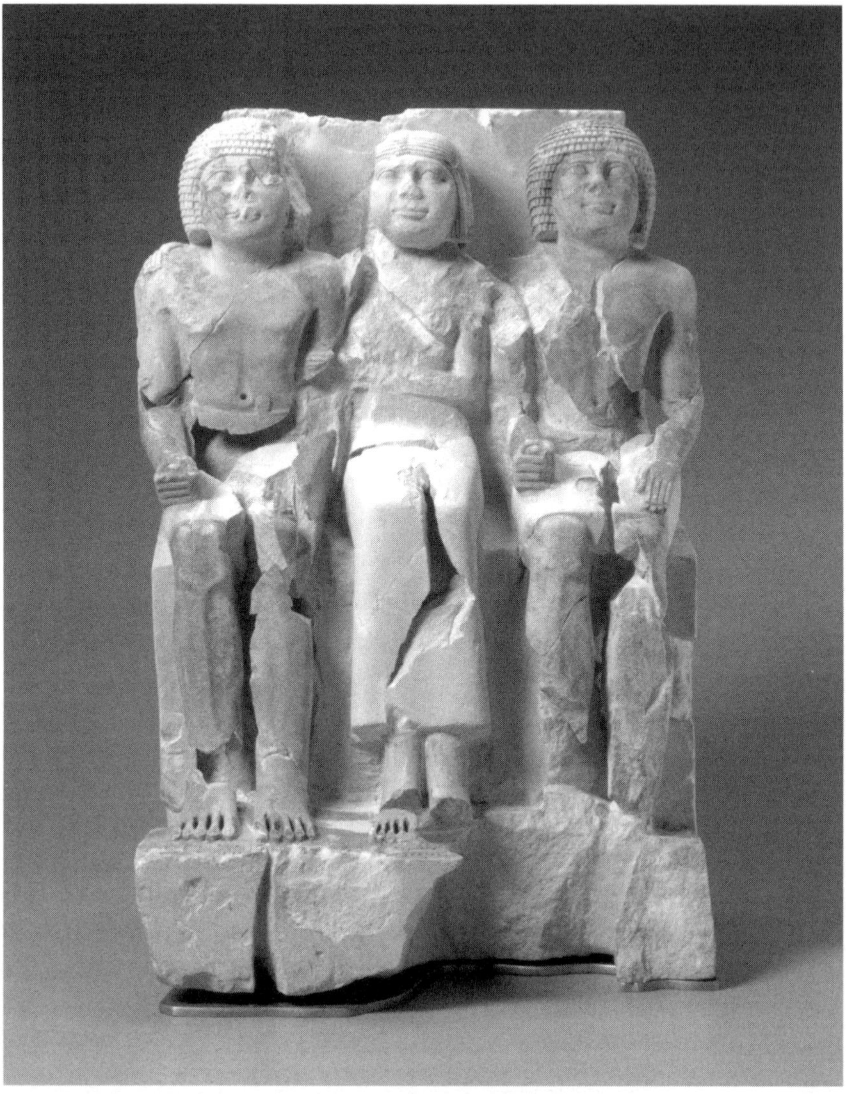

Fig. 4. Triad of Pehenptah and his mother. Egyptian, Old Kingdom, Fifth or Sixth Dynasty, 2465–2150 BC. Find-spot: Egypt, Giza, Tomb G 5280. Limestone. Overall: 25 3/8 × 16 15/16 × 16 in (64.5 × 43 × 40.6 cm). (Museum of Fine Arts, Boston, Harvard University—Boston Museum of Fine Arts Expedition, 13.4330.)

larly apparent in the case of the statue group of the dwarf Seneb and his (normal-sized) wife.[13] Both figures are shown seated. If realistic scale were maintained, that is, if isocephaly were not an important factor, Seneb would be shorter than his wife who was not a dwarf. However, to maintain equal height and status for Seneb, the sculptor has placed his figure on a pedestal, which raises him to the same level as his wife.

In some Old Kingdom sculpture, wives are much smaller than their husbands. This marked size difference between husband and wife seems to follow the principle of size dominance in which a more powerful figure is shown as significantly larger than other figures. In this type of depiction wives can be shown as half the size of their husbands.[14] A wife can also appear in statuary as a miniaturized version, perhaps serving the same function as a hieroglyphic inscription to indicate that the deceased was married. Size emphasizes the wife's dependent status.

The majority of preserved Egyptian art comes from tombs, and the compositional devices detailed above connect strongly to underlying beliefs about the nature of the universe. Scholars have long recognized that Egyptian art's "formulaic" quality reflects and in turn helps to construct a world view based on *maat*—the concept of a carefully balanced cosmos with pharaoh serving as guarantor. As Grzymski notes, pharaoh was "the key element of the society, not because of the political power of his office but because of his centrality to Egyptian ideology and religion. Without a king there would be no society to speak of, no state, and no order; there would only be chaos."[15] Tombs—the source of the best-preserved Egyptian art—were designed as microcosms of the established order. Funerary art provided the visual manifestation of this phenomenon, serving as a site that "associated earthly life processes of birth, maturation, parenthood and death with cosmic cycles and enduring time, thus formalizing the relationships between individuals and classes of individuals within

13. Statue of Seneb and family. Fifth Dynasty. Egyptian Museum Cairo. Malek, *Egypt: 4000 Years of Art*, Fig. 57.
14. Examples of smaller scale for wife: Pair Statue of Demedji and Henutsen. Metropolitan Museum of Art, New York, Rogers Fund, 1951 (51.37). D. Arnold, *When the Pyramids Were Built: Egyptian Art of the Old Kingdom* (New York: Rizzoli International Publications, 1999), Fig. 88; Wife as "hieroglyph": Statue of Ni-ka-re and his wife and daughter, Metropolitan Museum of Art New York, Rogers Fund, 1952. Arnold, *When the Pyramids Were Built*, Fig. 90. See also N. Cherpion, "The Human Image in Old Kingdom Nonroyal Reliefs," in *Egyptian Art in the Age of the Pyramids* (New York: Metropolitan Museum of Art, 1999), 112, for a discussion of this phenomenon in relief sculpture.
15. K. Grzymski, "Statuary," in *Egyptian Art in the Age of the Pyramids* (New York: Metropolitan Museum of Art, 1999), 51.

society."[16] Male/female, husband/wife were roles whose attributes were emphasized through images. Sculpture and writing provided a visual synopsis of the correct relations among elements of society.

Funerary sculpture is designed to depict an ideal view of society and to promote the correct relationships among humans and between humans and the divine, necessary to maintain *maat*. The emphasis in the sculptures and paintings that decorate Egyptian tombs is on the appropriateness and immutability of the social order. Thus, artistic depictions are not meant to indicate momentary states but rather the eternal essence of the object depicted. Sculptural images combine portraiture and the representational formulae. Size, color, and pose are all manipulated to produce an image that conforms to the correct social order. The images produced often appear quite lifelike; in fact, as Freed states, "Seldom was a statue an accurate portrait; rather it provided an ideal image of the way its owner wished to be remembered for eternity, regardless of actual age or appearance."[17] This emphasis on the ideal led to a restricted variety of ways in which figures could be shown. Baines coins an apt term for these restrictions when he labels them "decorum"—"a set of rules and practices defining what may be represented pictorially."[18] These formulae do not mimic nature so much as establish conformity to a world order that is promoted as "natural." Scale, costume, pose, and—as we shall see—color combine to support this world view rather than simply to imitate reality.

Women are never shown as anything but youthful and slender despite the fact that childbearing was one of their primary roles. Artistic images of women's costumes reveal much of the body underneath, suggesting a flimsy fabric. Yet in the rare actual finds of clothing from ancient Egypt the fabric is of much greater weight and thickness.[19] One can see a similar phenomenon at work in Classical Greek sculpture. The female figures of the East Pediment of the Parthenon wear costumes made of a "fantasy" fabric. The cloth is carved as if transparent in some areas and in others bunches up in thick, weighty folds.

Unlike women, men have more than one representational option, but a narrow range of types holds for them as well. Male figures can be shown as either

16. J. Lustig, "Kinship, Gender and Age in Middle Kingdom Tomb Scenes and Texts," in *Anthropology and Egyptology, A Developing Dialogue*, ed. J. Lustig (London: Sheffield, 1997), 63.
17. R. E. Freed, "Art," in *The Oxford Encyclopedia of Ancient Egypt*, ed. D. B. Redford (Oxford: Oxford University Press, 2001), Vol. 1, 128.
18. J. Baines, *Visual and Written Culture in Ancient Egypt*, 15.
19. Ibid., 17.

slender or with rolls of fat.[20] The extra weight indicates prosperity. The individual depicted has the wealth to acquire enough extra food to eat to get fat. Under such conditions, Tefnin observes, "naturalism does not mean realism."[21] True individualization was provided instead by the name painted or inscribed on the statue.[22] In this way the statue was a clear statement of the deceased's "adherence to a highly complex system of values known as *maat*, a cosmic principle of equilibrium."[23] Art supports and maintains a world view in which status and hierarchy as well as stability are very important. By reinforcing status differences—only the elite can commission pictorial representations—material culture promotes a world view in which pharaoh, supported by his court and government officials, holds his rightful place at the top of Egyptian society.[24]

The many artistic devices used to mark gender and gender roles described above indicate that the relationship between male and female forms an important element of the Egyptian world view. Art supports and shapes this aspect of Egyptian ideology. As I discuss in the Introduction, gender is a societal construct, not simply a reflection of nature, as cultural critics such as Judith Butler and Michel Foucault have shown. As Bahrani states, "gender is not a natural essence but something that is naturalised through repetition, through its societal inscription."[25] Male/female color differentiation, along with the other artistic rules that make up the Egyptian system of "decorum," was a way of "inscribing" the elite Egyptian view of gender relations.

Many indicators suggest that these gendered representations were deliberately imposed. The development of pharaonic rule was supported by a strongly controlled artistic program. Among these controls is the fact that artistic production is placed under the control of the state, and artists are trained in the canonical style. Even access to the materials used (hard stone, wood, precious metals, etc.) was under the king's control.[26] Cult statues, temple decorations for the gods, and images to house the spirits of the deceased throughout the afterlife were used as vehicles to convey pharaoh's message. While scholars have in-

20. See for example the Old Kingdom statue of Hemiunu. Roemer- und Pelizaeus-Museum, Hildesheim 19620. D. Arnold, *When the Pyramids Were Built: Egyptian Art of the Old Kingdom*, Fig. 33.
21. R. Tefnin, "Sculpture: Private Sculpture," in D. B. Redford, *The Oxford Encyclopedia of Ancient Egypt*, Vol. 3, 241.
22. R. Freed, "Art," in Redford, *The Oxford Encyclopedia of Ancient Egypt*, Vol. 1, 128.
23. D. Spanel, *Through Ancient Eyes: Egyptian Portraiture* (Birmingham, AL: The Museum, 1988), 6.
24. On this point see J. Baines, *Visual and Written Culture in Ancient Egypt*, 14.
25. Z. Bahrani, *Women of Babylon: Gender and Representation in Mesopotamia* (London: Routledge, 2001), 32.
26. On this point see A. Kozloff, "Sculpture: An Overview," in D. B. Redford, *The Oxford Encyclopedia of Ancient Egypt*, Vol. 3, 218.

tensely studied the Roman use of art in the service of the state, other than for the Amarna period scholars have generally not recognized "pharaonic agency" in the creation of Egyptian art. That Augustus, the first Roman emperor, could manipulate art to legitimize his rule is a scholarly given.[27] It seems no less likely that the earliest unifiers of Egypt would have done the same thing. Rice points to a "powerful, united and supremely well-focused elite" as the catalyst for such a deliberate iconographical program.[28] The artistic program supports and reinforces elite status.

An important component of this program was the articulation of the status and role of women within Egyptian society. Egyptian literature reveals that a consistent theme in the maintenance of *maat* is unity achieved through the union of opposites that complement each other. The union of male and female was an important component of the desired balance and harmony in the universe. The sun itself was reborn each day through the union of the setting sun (male) and the earth (female). The emphasis on correct world order in Egyptian art suggests that color differentiation should in some way reflect a view of the relationship between male and female that supports and upholds that order. Color, like the other stylistic features discussed above, is part of a complex symbolic system. It marks women as separate from men.

How then does male/female color differentiation fit into the Egyptian world view exemplified by *maat*? Like Classical Archaeologists, some Egyptologists have embraced the traditional explanation that male/female color differentiation reflects a natural difference in sun exposure between women, whose lives were conducted indoors, and men, whose lives were focused outside the house.[29] Other scholars have suggested that male/female color differentiation may hold a deeper symbolic meaning.[30] As Robins states, "the colors given to human skin—although initially seeming to be naturalistic—might also be symbolic."[31] An examination of the history of Egyptian male/female color differentiation will shed some light on this debate.

By the Fourth Dynasty, usually considered the beginning of the Old King-

---

27. On Augustus see P. Zanker, *The Power of Images in the Age of Augustus* (Ann Arbor: University of Michigan Press, 1988).
28. M. Rice, *Egypt's Making: The Origins of Ancient Egypt (5000–2000 B.C.)* (London: Routledge, 2003), 72.
29. See for example J. Malek, *Egypt: 4000 Years of Art*, 46, and R. H. Wilkinson, *Symbol and Magic in Egyptian Art*, 115.
30. See for example G. Robins, "Gender Roles," in Redford, *The Oxford Encyclopedia of Ancient Egypt*, Vol. 2, 12–16, and J. Tydesley, *Chronicles of the Queens of Egypt* (London: Thames and Hudson, 2006), 12.
31. G. Robins, "Color Symbolism," in Redford, *The Oxford Encyclopedia of Ancient Egypt*, Vol. 1, 292.

dom, there is a codification and stabilization of kingly power and its iconography. Color, just as are scale and position, is part of a consistent program of representation that reflects the Egyptian ruling elite's view of status and power and reflects underlying gender roles amplified during the shift to pharaonic rule. It is no surprise then that the best preserved early examples of male/female color differentiation in Egyptian art belong to this period.[32] Many other features considered typical of Egyptian art—such as an emphasis on frontality in freestanding sculpture and profile views for human figures in relief sculpture—are also formalized by this period. Male/female color differentiation appears in freestanding statues and in relief sculpture. Men are painted a dark reddish-brown, women a lighter shade—white, tan, cream, or yellow. Figure 5, the Fifth Dynasty seated statue of Rahotep and his wife Nofret from Rahotep's tomb chapel at Meidum (ca. 2550 BC),[33] is a very clear example of this use of color. Rahotep's skin is painted a dark brown and Nofret's a light cream. Color differentiation is an added feature to distinguish male from female. The two figures would be identifiable as a man and a woman without this color treatment; they are also differentiated by costume and hairstyle, as well as by secondary sexual characteristics. He wears a kilt and has short hair and a moustache. She wears a skintight long white sheath, a decorated pectoral, and a headdress over shoulder-length hair.

That color differentiation was standard practice in the Old Kingdom can be seen from numerous examples. I will describe only the best-known examples, but the pattern holds for most Old Kingdom sculpture and painting. The Fifth Dynasty statue group of the dwarf Seneb and his family from Giza[34] shows an even sharper contrast in skin tones between male and female than does Rahotep and Nofret's statue. The skin of Seneb's wife is white, while Seneb's is dark reddish-brown. Their children, carved in relief as miniatures on the front of the statue's pedestal, are depicted as prepubescent nudes. The skin of the girl is painted white like her mother's and the skin of the boy dark reddish-brown like his father's. In the Fifth Dynasty family group of Sekedkau, husband and wife

32. Examples include Pair Statue of Katep and Hetep-Heres, Painted Limestone, Trustees of the British Museum, London EA 1181. D. Arnold, K. Grzymski, and C. Ziegler, eds., *Egyptian Art in the Age of the Pyramids* (New York: Metropolitan Museum of Art, 1999), Catalogue No. 82, 290; Pair Statue of Iai-ib and Khuaut 30.8 cm, Ägyptisches Museum, Universität Leipzig 3684, Arnold, Grzymski, and Ziegler 1999, Catalogue No. 83, 293. Neither the state of preservation nor our ability to precisely date Old Kingdom sculpture allows any one piece to be labeled the first example of male/female color differentiation. It is, however, an established practice by the Fourth Dynasty.

33. G. Robins, *The Art of Ancient Egypt* (Cambridge: Cambridge University Press, 1997), Fig. 51.

34. Statue of Seneb. Cairo, Egyptian Museum. Malek, *Egypt: 4000 Years of Art*, Fig. 57.

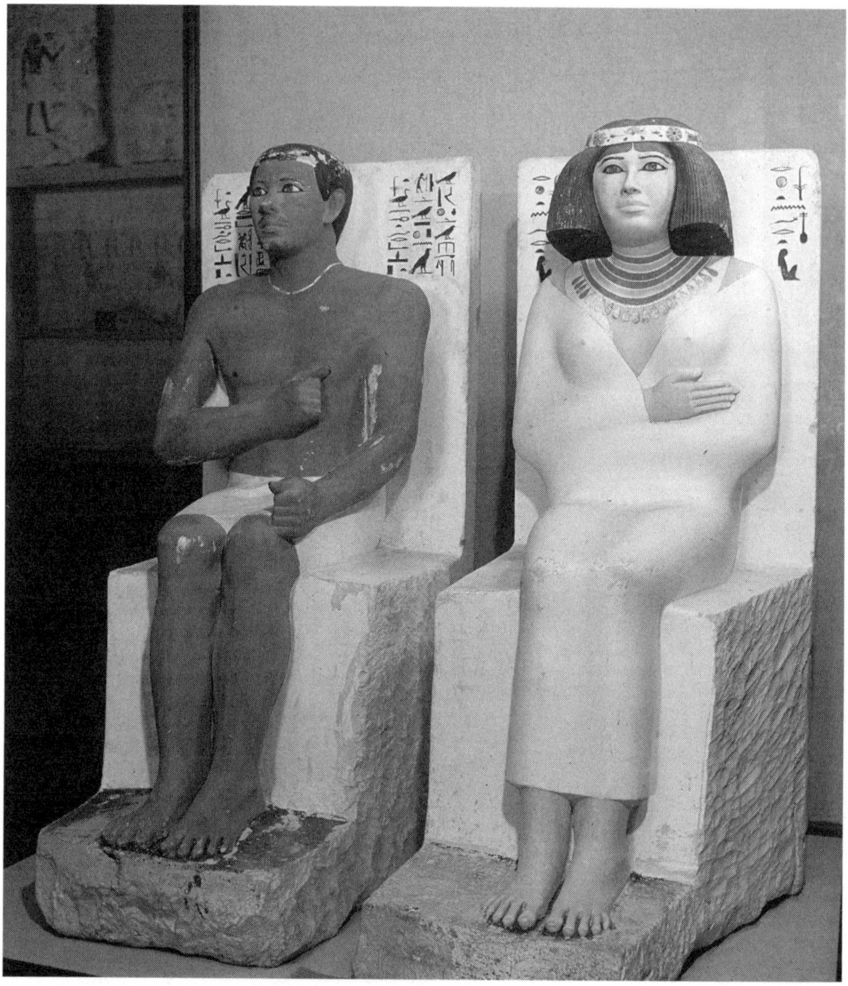

Fig. 5. Statues of Prince Rahotep and his wife Nofret. Nofret's jewelery, costume, and wig are vividly portrayed. 4th dynasty—ca. 2613–2944 BC. Painted limestone H.121 cm. (From Maidum, Egyptian Museum, Cairo, Egypt. Photo Credit: Werner Forman/Art Resource, NY.)

are shown seated with their son standing to the wife's right.[35] Again they are also differentiated by costume. Both males wear kilts, while the female figure wears a long white sleeveless tunic decorated above the waist with a pattern of horizontal lines and scallops. Father and son are both shown with dark-reddish-brown flesh, while Sekedkau's wife's flesh is painted a light tan. The pattern is repeated in a statue of Katep and his wife Hetepheres from Giza, also Fifth Dynasty.[36] She wears a tunic similar to the one described above and he wears a kilt. His flesh is a bright reddish-brown and hers a light yellow.

These examples show that contrasting skin tone is not simply a method of distinguishing between men and women in a group or pair. The dark/light convention is maintained even when a single figure rather than a couple is depicted. Princess Nefertiabet is shown alone on a Fourth Dynasty slab stela from Giza.[37] Her skin is painted yellow. On the slab stele from the Saqqara (Second Dynasty) a male tomb owner is shown alone, and his skin is painted the typical dark-reddish-brown male color.[38]

All of the examples of male/female color differentiation discussed thus far have been depictions from the tombs of elite men and women. Before the Sixth Dynasty a tomb with its attendant sculptural decoration was a special sign of favor granted by pharaoh and restricted to the Egyptian elite—members of the court and the administration.[39] The question remains as to whether color differentiation is used in depictions of lower-class individuals. The absence of male/female color differentiation in non-elite images might suggest that color differentiation could be used not just to distinguish male from female but to distinguish elite men and women from the lower classes. However, whether color differentiation functioned in this way is not easy to determine since there are not many clearly identifiable images of the lower classes to examine. During the Old Kingdom tombs are equipped with stone statues of individuals performing everyday tasks such as baking and brewing. These sculptures were traditionally identified by scholars as "servant statues" and consequently considered depictions of non-elite individuals.[40]

A prominent group, the largest preserved from any single tomb, consists of

---

35. Cairo Museum CG 101. R. Bianchi, *Splendors of Ancient Egypt* (London: Booth-Clibborn, 1996), Figs. 52 and 53.
36. London British Museum. G. Robins, *The Art of Ancient Egypt*, Fig. 69.
37. From Giza. Louvre, Paris. Malek, *Egypt: 4000 Years of Art*, Fig. 56.
38. From Saqarra (Second Dynasty). G. Robins, *The Art of Ancient Egypt*, Fig. 35.
39. D. Spanel, *Through Ancient Eyes: Egyptian Portraiture* (Birmingham, AL: The Museum, 1988), 11.
40. The standard work is J. H. Breasted, *Egyptian Servant Statues* (New York: Pantheon Books, 1948).

twenty-five figures from the tomb of Ny-Kau-Inpu, a cemetery official of the Fifth Dynasty.[41] The sculptures depict individuals preparing bread and beer and butchering oxen and fowl, the traditional foodstuffs given as offerings to the deceased. Among the figurines male and female are clearly differentiated by the standard colors. This would then be an indication that non-elite men and women were depicted with the same artistic device as their elite counterparts. However, recent studies have suggested that these figurines may not represent "actual" servants but the relatives of the deceased providing the necessary nourishment for the afterlife and perhaps ensuring their own afterlife by accompanying the deceased in this symbolic form.[42] The statues from Ny-Kau-Inpu's tomb support this assertion since short hieroglyphic inscriptions identify the statues as family members, although the lack of inscriptions on similar statues from other tombs makes it difficult to know if this was always the case.

Figures traditionally described by scholars as servants are also shown in relief sculpture from Old Kingdom tombs. The deceased is shown in larger scale supervising the "servants." Unlike the figures described above there are no inscriptions identifying these figures as family members. Dark/light color differentiation is used for these figures, and if the lack of other identification does indeed indicate that the figures are servants we can identify these figures as non-elite men and women. The consistent use of male/female color differentiation for these figures would tend to discount social class as one of the factors associated with color differentiation.

Color differentiation also holds true for representations of pharaoh. A dark diorite statue of King Menkaure (Fourth Dynasty) and his queen preserves traces of red paint on his skin and yellow on hers.[43] Even gods and goddesses are distinguished in this way (Fig. 6). In a relief of King Snefru, also from the Fourth Dynasty, the king is shown with the lion-headed goddess Sekhmet. King Snefru's skin is the traditional reddish brown, and Sekhmet's is the same light color reserved for mortal females.[44] However, a more specialized color symbolism is associated with male deities.[45] While they are usually painted the

41. For this group of statues see E. Teeter, *Ancient Egypt: Treasures from the Collection of the Oriental Institute* (Chicago: University of Chicago, 1999), Catalogue No. 137.
42. M. Hill, "Dwarf Musician," in Arnold, Ziegler, and Roehrig, eds., *Egyptian Art in the Age of the Pyramids*, 389.
43. King Menkaure and a Queen. Museum of Fine Arts Boston, Harvard University-Museum of Fine Arts Expedition (11.1738). Arnold, Ziegler, and Roehrig, eds., *Egyptian Art in the Age of the Pyramids*, Fig. on p. 50, Cat. No. 67.
44. G. Robins, *The Art of Ancient Egypt*, Fig. 44, p. 49.
45. B. Bryan, "In Women Good and Bad Fortune Are on Earth: Status and Roles of Women in Egyptian

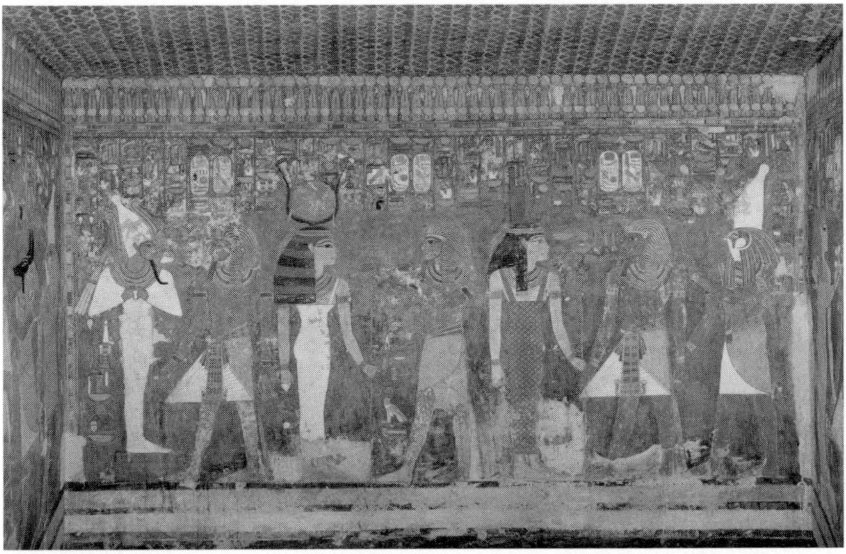

Fig. 6. Mural painting in the burial chamber. Pharaoh before Osiris, Isis, Ma'at, and Horus. (Photo: S. Vannini. Tomb of Harehmheb, Valley of the Kings, Thebes, Egypt. © DeA Picture Library/Art Resource, NY.)

same reddish-brown color used for mortal men, certain gods are given other skin colors because of their spheres of influence. For example, the skin of Osiris is often painted black or green because of his association with rebirth through the fertility of the earth. In these cases the use of color is clearly symbolic. This again raises the question of whether the standard male/female convention is also symbolic. That is the question which was the initial stimulus and focus for this book—Is the dark/light convention a realistic depiction of actual difference between men and women, or does it reflect a deeper symbolic meaning?

Discovering a deeper symbolic meaning is not an easy task since in Egyptian art color is used in different ways depending upon context. In some situations color was used "realistically." On the one hand, objects were painted the color that they appear in nature—green for plants, blue for sky. On the other hand, objects could be painted colors that had symbolic rather than "realistic" connotations. For example, green could be used to depict plants, a "realistic"

Culture," in A. Capel and G. Markoe, eds., *Mistress of the House, Mistress of Heaven: Women in Ancient Egypt*, 35. R. H. Wilkinson, *Symbol and Magic in Egyptian Art*, 113.

use, but the sickle that was used to cut plants was also painted green, symbolizing its connection to the fertility of the harvest.

Attempting to discriminate between the symbolic and realistic uses of color becomes particularly difficult when dealing with skin color. As noted above, the skin of the gods is usually depicted according to the male/female color convention, but there are many instances in which other colors are used. The skin of gods is often painted in a symbolic hue. Osiris is shown with black skin, connecting him with the "renewing" properties of Egypt's "black soil" as part of his role as underworld deity associated with the rebirth that the Egyptians believed occurred in the afterlife. Using this same symbolic motif, black stone came to signify rebirth when used in sculpture.[46] Blue could be used for the sky but also for the skin of divinities as an indication of their high status, since the color represented lapis lazuli. Green could also be used for the skin color of gods associated with abundance, suggesting an association with plant life and perhaps life-giving water.[47] Does male/female color differentiation belong to the natural category of color designations such as the use of green for reeds and grasses or to a more symbolic system, like the black flesh of Osiris?

Any discussion of symbolic versus realistic skin color must examine the question of what the "actual" skin color of ancient Egyptians was. As Robins points out:

> Male and female skin colors were most probably not uniform among the entire population of Egypt, with pigmentation being darker in the South (closer to sub-Saharan Africans) and lighter in the North (closer to Mediterranean Near Easterners). A woman from the South would probably have had darker skin than a man from the North.[48]

This question of "actual" skin color is deeply mired in discussions about race, which have more to do with our own society's history and values than with those of ancient Egypt. Early scholarship sought to distance Egypt from black Africa, and textbooks often showed Egyptians as "white."[49] Scholars of the early twentieth century considered the Egyptians a "brown" race.[50] More recently,

46. G. Robins "Color Symbolism," in D. B. Redford, *The Oxford Encyclopedia of Ancient Egypt*, Vol. 1, 291.
47. R. H. Wilkinson, *Symbol and Magic in Egyptian Art*, 122.
48. G. Robins, "Color Symbolism," in Redford, *The Oxford Encyclopedia of Ancient Egypt*, Vol. 1, 293.
49. S. T. Smith "Race," in Redford, *The Oxford Encyclopedia of Ancient Egypt*, Vol. 3, 111–16.
50. See for example J. H. Breasted, *The Conquest of Civilization* (New York: HarperCollins, 1926), revised edition 1938, 43.

Afro-centric scholarship seeks to make Egyptians "black."[51] While modern anthropological studies have shown that race is more of a sociological construct than a biological absolute, these discussions persist.[52] For Egypt, as Cheal has shown, there is no evidence of an emphasis on racial purity or legal status based on ethnic origin.[53]

Scenes from Eighteenth Dynasty tombs of Huy and Sbekhotep and the Nineteenth Dynasty tombs of Ramses III and Sety I show that the Egyptians could use skin color to differentiate among different ethnic groups.[54] For example, in the Nineteenth Dynasty tombs that depict a group of subject peoples (all male) offering tribute to pharaoh, the Nubians are shown with black skin, the Near Easterners with yellow, and the Libyans with white. However, each group is also clearly marked by its distinctive hairstyle and clothing. Skin color is not the only distinctive feature. Skin color is not used to set up a hierarchy analogous to the American racial model, a lingering and reprehensible legacy of slavery, in which light skin is accorded higher status than dark. In fact, Libyans, Bedouins, Syrians, and Hittites, while differentiated by costume in groups of subject peoples, are all painted the lighter color reserved for women in gender differentiation. If the American racial value system were in fact in place, the conquered Nubians would have a higher status than the conquering Egyptians since their skin is the lightest. Instead the crucial factor in distinguishing these groups is to show the diversity of foreigners over which pharaoh has control. Their variety stresses the enormity of his task and thus his success. His continued control against these various forces, usually described as chaotic and uncivilized, guarantees the universe.[55] Color is again used symbolically rather than realistically.

Support for the realistic use of color in male/female color differentiation does, at first glance, seem to be found in a few exceptional instances in Old and Middle Kingdom painting in which the freshly shaved heads of men are painted

---

51. C. A. Diop, *The African Origins of Civilization* (Chicago: Lawrence Hill Books, 1974).
52. K. Viswerseram, "Race and the Culture of Anthropology," *American Anthropologist* 100 (1998): 70–83. See also F. Snowden, *Before Color Prejudice* (Cambridge: Harvard University Press, 1983), for a discussion of ancient views on race.
53. C. Cheal, "The Meaning of Skin Color in Eighteenth Dynasty Egypt," in *Race and Identity in the Nile Valley*, ed. C. Fluehr-Lobban and K. Rhodes, 54.
54. Ramses II: Polychrome Faience Foreign Captives. Funerary Temple of Ramses III. Medinet Habu. Egypt Cairo Museum. J. Malek, *Egypt: 4000 Years of Art*. See also C. Cheal, "The Meaning of Skin Color in Eighteenth Dynasty Egypt," in *Race and Identity in the Nile Valley*, 58. Tomb of Sety I. Four Races of Humankind. Valley of the Kings, Thebes. Nineteenth Dynasty. R. H. Wilkinson, *Symbol and Magic in Egyptian Art*, Fig. 82, p. 115.
55. On this point see G. Robins, "Color Symbolism," in D. B. Redford, *The Oxford Encyclopedia of Ancient Egypt*, Vol. 1, 293.

yellow—a color usually reserved for female flesh—while the remainder of their bodies is the typical reddish-brown color. Fischer suggests that this difference in color indicates that the yellow area on top of these figures' heads had previously been protected from the sun by the now-shaved hair.[56] These are anomalous figures and difficult to explain. In this case, red/yellow color differentiation does seem to be tied to sun exposure. Since Egyptian art usually stresses permanent rather than temporary states, however, the shaved heads must have had a particular significance that caused this feature to be marked by the artist.

There are also several Old Kingdom examples of men with yellow flesh (a typical female flesh color) that some argue indicate that male/female color differentiation is a result of differences in sun exposure between men and women. The men in these yellow-skinned representations are almost all shown as very heavy with pendulous breasts.[57] The pale skin color and heaviness of the individuals could suggests a sedentary and thus indoor existence. One could also argue for a symbolic interpretation. Yellow older men could indicate a diminution in power that would make these men equivalent to women who, as we shall see, had a lesser political status than men. Another possibility suggested by Cheal is that this skin color choice is representative of light colors of metal such as gold and silver that can be linked with aging in a positive light, namely, divine aging. A New Kingdom tomb tells a story about Amun-Re that describes him as "old" with gold flesh. The yellow flesh would thus connect these older men to divine immortality.[58] If, however, the skin of these men is meant to be "gold," it would be a conflation of the color yellow with the precious metal, which as noted above does not usually occur even for images of the gods, whose flesh is sometimes described as gold but shown in the colors of male/female color differentiation. Another possible conflation would be the connection of Hathor, who is most often described as the "Golden goddess" with the yellow used for female skin color. This would be an added layer of meaning for this color use.[59] The uniqueness of these yellow Egyptian males points to the fact that color is not always used in a clearly readable (at least by us) fashion.

A factor that has largely been overlooked in discussions of these anomalously colored male figures is that similar anomalies do not occur for women

---

56. For examples see H. G. Fischer, "Varia Aegyptiaca 1. Yellow-Skinned Representations of Men in the Old Kingdom," *Journal of the American Research Center in Egypt* 2 (1963): 17–22.
57. Ibid.
58. C. Cheal, "The Meaning of Skin Color in Eighteenth Dynasty Egypt," in *Race and Identity in the Nile Valley*, 63.
59. Ibid., 63.

(with the exception, as we shall see in Chapter 2, of the New Kingdom reigns of Hatshepsut and Akhenaten). Women shown working in the fields—and thus outside in the sun—have the typical yellow female color, not the reddish brown that one might expect if color were a reflection of outdoor activity.[60] This suggests that as far as women were concerned a symbolic meaning is taking precedence over a "realistic" depiction. These depictions also militate against the idea that pale skin color is a marker solely of elite status for women. If that were the case one might expect that upper-class women would deliberately accentuate lighter skin, yet there is no evidence that elite Egyptian women used cosmetics for skin lightening.[61] It is apparently more important for the sculpture to emphasize that the figures are female than that they are outdoors. Indeed, preserved hieratic lists of people used by schoolmasters organize by gender first and then by class and nationality.[62]

As we have seen from the examples of yellow male figures, males can be shown in either a symbolic or "realistic" manner. Male divinities also exhibit greater flexibility in skin colors. As discussed earlier, they can be shown with skin painted colors other than the traditional reddish brown. Yet the skin of goddesses almost never deviates from the conventional colors used for mortal women. This greater variety in depiction for mortal and divine males compared with mortal and divine females extends, as we shall see later in this chapter, to other aspects of representational art, including the types of statues that are available for men and women. The male principle is always emphasized through greater range of types and greater variety in portrayal.

These types of distinctions further support the idea that male/female color differentiation is not simply a matter of relative sun exposure. The fact that a wider variety of skin color options is given to male figures suggests that color may be used in a symbolic fashion to support a dominant role for men in society. Restriction in the range of colors for female figures dovetails with the narrower range of statue types available to mortal women and also fits in with their generally more restricted roles in government, which I will discuss in more detail below. Once again art serves to emphasize status. Color supports this "iconography of power."

---

60. See for example the Eighteenth Dynasty harvesting scene from the Tomb of Nakht (Thebes No. 52). A. Mekhitarian, *Egyptian Painting* (New York: Rizzoli, 1978), 73. C. Cheal, "The Meaning of Skin Color in Eighteenth Dynasty Egypt," in *Race and Identity in the Nile Valley*, 59.
61. C. Cheal, "The Meaning of Skin Color in Eighteenth Dynasty Egypt," 59.
62. Ibid., 60. A. Erman, *Ancient Egyptian Poetry and Prose*, trans. A. Blackman (New York: Dover, 1995 [1923]), 187.

However, the same dark/light, yellow/red, or red/white color contrast can also be used in what appears to be a non-realistic and a non-symbolic fashion. Because the depth of relief is so low in Old Kingdom sculpture, the same color difference used to distinguish male and female is used to differentiate overlapping men in depictions of lines of men, and a lighter shade of brown is used to distinguish between two combatants in wrestling. By alternating traditionally male reddish brown with traditionally female white or yellow, the artist eliminates confusion over where one figure ends and another begins. Alternating colors, although not the standard male/female colors, are also used to differentiate one animal from another in overlapping files.[63] In these cases color would seem to function as a purely formal artistic device and not in a symbolic manner. There might, however, be more going on in the case of the wrestlers. They appear in the tomb of Amenmose (ca. 1300 BC).[64] Several contesting pairs are shown involved in stick fighting and wrestling. In each case the combatant who seems to be losing is painted a lighter color than the victor, although not the yellow or white color of women. This light skin could suggest lesser, that is, "feminine," strength.

Further complexity is introduced when one looks for literary symbolism associated with the particular colors used for male/female color differentiation—reddish brown, white, and yellow. The Egyptians regarded color as a sign of an object's true nature. The connection between the nature of a figure and its color is emphasized by the fact that Egyptian words for "color" and "character" are identical, indicating that the underlying essence of a figure can be expressed through color.[65] Male/female color differentiation would thus function as a symbolic statement of the essence or character of female and male.

However, Egyptian texts attest to only four color terms. These terms roughly translate into English as *black*, *white*, *green* (which may also have included blue), and *red*. These terms included within them colors that the European system of color designation would consider distinct. The Egyptian term for red, for example, also included yellow and orange. Red in Egyptian art is usually closer to our "brown" and yellow is ochre colored.[66] On the other hand, the

63. H. Schäfer, *Principles of Egyptian Art*, epilogue by Emma Brunner-Traut; translated and edited with an Introduction by John Baines (Oxford: Griffith Institute, 1974), 78. See, for example, The Tomb of Menna (Thebes No. 69). Mekhitarian, *Egyptian Painting*, 76.

64. Tomb of Amenmose (T 19) Dra abu'l Naga. C. K. Wilkinson and M. Hill, *Egyptian Wall Paintings*, 32.61, Fig. 36. On these figures see also N. Marinatos, *Art and Religion in Thera* (Athens: D & I Mathioulakis, 1984), 77.

65. J. Baines, *Visual and Written Culture in Ancient Egypt*, 244.

66. J. Baines, *Fecundity Figures* (Chicago: Griffith Institute, 1985), 289.

colors visible in Old Kingdom tomb paintings are more numerous. The preserved color palette, derived from ground minerals, consists of black, white, red, green, yellow, blue, and gray. While gold is also a prominent color, the word for gold belonged to the vocabulary of precious metals rather than to color terms. Some minerals such as lapis lazuli followed a similar pattern; although the mineral was blue it was described as a precious stone rather than as a color. Art thus shows a greater color repertoire than language. Visual vocabulary took precedence over written terminology. As Baines notes, "Color [in Egypt] is more easily painted than talked about."[67] We cannot rely upon texts to describe meanings attributed to specific colors because the terminology does not specify all of the shades found in art. Artistic usage sometimes contradicts the literary. For example, the flesh of the gods is described in texts as "gold" (not a term for color or shade but the word for the precious metal).[68] In art, however, the skin of the gods is painted with the same male/female color convention used for mortals. This suggests that the binary opposition of male and female takes precedence over the divinity of the subjects depicted. Even when the goddess Sekhmet is shown with the head of a lion, her human limbs are painted the yellow color reserved for females. Male gods are painted the dark-reddish-brown male color.

Examining the contexts in which different colors appear makes it possible to see whether male/female skin color differentiation harmonizes with any underlying themes in Egyptian ideology. Two emerge as particularly relevant—complementarity and completion expressed through dualities.[69] In the Egyptian world view various pairings were used to express unity. For example, the country was called the "two lands," and many motifs reflecting this unity, such as northern and southern figures binding the plants of the region, were shown. This motif was a symbolic representation of a much more complex political development, the unification of the country under pharaonic rule. Once unification was in place, a wide-ranging and powerful symbolism evolved that required double rituals for kingship and cult. Most of the ceremonies of kingship—coronation, jubilee activities, and so forth—were presented in double form. The king is often shown presenting two identical offerings to the gods. Wilkinson suggests that "this duality must have meant much more to the an-

67. Ibid.
68. R. H. Wilkinson, *Symbol and Magic in Egyptian Art*, 83.
69. J. Tydesley, *Chronicles of the Queens of Egypt*, 12. R. H. Wilkinson, *Symbol and Magic in Egyptian Art*, 141, 154. E. S. Meltzer, "Who Knows the Color of God?" *Journal of Ancient Civilizations* 11 (1996): 125.

cient Egyptians than merely the celebration of united dual kingdoms, for it was based upon and thus affirmed the nature of the creation itself and characterized the fundamental aspects of the universe."[70]

Complementary dualities reflected not only the north-south orientation of the Nile but also the belief in a dichotomy between the physical and the spiritual. The Egyptians often formed dualities by linking opposites. As Wilkinson notes, the world was divided into "pairs by which aspects of reality were labeled and which often describe the world in terms of the opposite yet complementary aspects of stasis and change."[71] Among the gods, Osiris, who symbolized stability, was often paired with Seth, who embodied chaos. Other oppositional pairs include the earth, which is characterized as male, and the sky, which is characterized as female.

Male/female color differentiation could emphasize the fact that man and woman are also an oppositional duality. The colors chosen for male and female skin color are the key elements in indicating that men and women are opposites. In Egyptian thought red (which encompasses brown) and white often functioned as symbolic opposites. Yellow, for which there is no separate color term, is also often substituted for white. Egyptian color symbolism allows for a transfer of properties from one color to another, and this is particularly common between yellow and white. Thus yellow, like white, could serve as an opposite to red.[72]

While opposition between red and white/yellow is important, the main feature of any duality in Egyptian ideology is the *combination* of the two opposing elements. Examples of this pairing include the red and white crowns used to signify Osiris (stability) and Seth (chaos). Together they symbolized the order of the universe as well as the unification of Upper and Lower Egypt. For the Egyptians such unions of opposites symbolized completion.[73] For example, the creator god Atum's name means both "totality" and "not to be," thus combining within himself the opposing states of existence and non-existence.[74] This duality finds expression in the two crowns of Egypt—the white crown of Upper Egypt and the red crown of Lower Egypt.

---

70. R. H. Wilkinson, *Symbol and Magic in Egyptian Art*, 130.
71. Ibid., 129.
72. On yellow see J. Baines, *Fecundity Figures*, 86, and J. Baines, *Visual and Written Culture in Ancient Egypt*, 247. On the transferral between the two colors see R. H. Wilkinson, *Symbol and Magic in Egyptian Art*, 111.
73. R. H. Wilkinson, *Symbol and Magic in Egyptian Art*, 112.
74. On Atum see V. A. Tobin, "Creation Myths," in D. B. Redford, *The Oxford Encyclopedia of Ancient Egypt*, Vol. 1, 469.

In such a world view the contrasting color system of male/female color differentiation emphasizes the symbolic completion embodied in uniting the opposites of male and female. It does not serve simply to contrast degrees of sun exposure, especially since both colors can also be associated with solar imagery. While red could be used to signify the intense radiance of the sun (red was used for amulets of the "Eye of Re," the sun god),[75] the color we identify as yellow was also connected with the sun. Statues made of red or yellow stone were used for images of pharaohs who wished to be equated with the sun god. Clear differentiation between male and female was particularly important in asserting the reproductive spheres the Egyptians associated with each sex. These reproductive roles serve a vital function in Egyptian funerary ideology. *Maat* (world order) was maintained by the union of male and female. The union of male and female takes on even greater significance in the context of the afterlife where women were necessary as the catalyst for reproduction, which, in turn, guaranteed the afterlife.[76]

The role of woman as catalyst is clearly seen in Egyptian cosmologies. In the Egyptian cosmology the act of creation was literally in the hands of the male god Re-Atum. There are several versions but, as the Old Kingdom Pyramid texts state, "Atum is he who (once) came into being who masturbated in On. He took his phallus in his grasp that he might create orgasm by means of it, and so were born the twins Shu and Tefenet."[77] An alternate cosmology from coffin texts of the Middle Kingdom also attributes the act of creation to the male, this time Nun, the primeval water, who produces four pairs of male and female deities.[78]

Thus Creation was centered on a male god. In the human realm, as well, the male was seen as the locus of fertility. The female was the catalyst for stimulating male fertility. As Roth states, "The responsibility for fertility and creating new life was not laid on the shoulders of women in ancient Egypt, they were instead expected to be sexually aggressive, to begin the process of creation by enticing their male partners to creation."[79] This view extends from the divine

75. R. H. Wilkinson, *Symbol and Magic in Egyptian Art*, 107.
76. G. Robins, "Dress, Undress and the Representation of Fertility and Potency in New Kingdom Egyptian Art," in N. B. Kampen, ed., *Sexuality in Ancient Art* (Cambridge: Cambridge University Press, 1996), 27–40.
77. R. O. Faulkner, *The Ancient Egyptian Pyramid Texts* (Oxford: Oxford University Press, 1969), 1248.
78. F. Hassan, "Earliest Goddesses of Egypt: Divine Mothers and Cosmic Bodies," in *Ancient Goddesses, The Myths and the Evidence*, ed. L. Goodison and C. Morris (Madison: University of Wisconsin Press, 1998), 107.
79. A. M. Roth, "Father Earth, Mother Sky: Ancient Egyptian Beliefs about Conception and Fertility," in

sphere where the hand with which Atum masturbated and thus began the process of creation was personified as a goddess. Such stimulation was a guarantee of the afterlife. As Cheal has shown, red can be associated with this creative power since Atum and also the sun god Re were sometimes portrayed as red. She further suggests that images of a red fish, the tilapia, can be used to represent the phallus and thereby symbolize male fertility, since the male holds the eggs in its mouth until they hatch, thus giving birth to the young.[80]

Many of the motifs found in tomb paintings show women in situations that indicate their role as catalysts. The female body is the focus for stimulation of the male in the afterlife. As early as the Sixth Dynasty, tombs include the motif of the owner's wife playing the harp on the marital bed, an image suggestive of the sexual activity necessary for rebirth. Recent studies of banquet scenes in tombs suggest that there is a strong sexual element in these seemingly quotidian scenes.[81] Robins suggests that the tight costume depicted on Old Kingdom images of elite women is also designed to emphasize female sexuality. Males, on the other hand, wear kilts, which never reveal any hint of the genitals. This emphasis on the role of women as stimulator of the sexual union necessary for the afterlife may explain the fact that the majority of statues of women come from funerary contexts. While statues of men are found in temples and shrines as well as tombs, the majority of statues of women are found only in tombs. Men's other roles were stressed in statues found in other contexts, but women were presented in the afterlife in the specific role of sexual catalyst.[82]

Male/female color differentiation marks the difference in spheres of activity between men and women, but also emphasizes that the combination of these two opposites, brought together in sexual union, provides for the afterlife and maintains the stable order of the universe. Male and female serve as "complementary sources of generation, which make possible the continuing process of

Reading the Body: Representations and Remains in the Archaeological Record, ed. A. Rautman (Philadelphia: University of Pennsylvania Press, 2000), 200.

80. C. Cheal, "The Meaning of Skin Color in Eighteenth Dynasty Egypt," in *Race and Identity in the Nile Valley*, 62. Although interesting, this interpretation may be incorrect in that the actual Egyptian Mouthbreeder (*Pseudocrenilabrus multicolor*) is actually a maternal mouthbrooder. The Black-chinned Tilapia (*Sarotherodon melanotheron*) is one of the few paternal mouthbrooders, but its range is primarily the west coast of Africa (T. M. Kalk, G. Teugels, and E. Abban, "Revision and Biographical Analysis of the Black-chinned Tilapia," *Journal of Natural History*, [2002]: 2191–2212).

81. On this point see L. Manniche, "Sexuality," in D. Redford, *The Oxford Encyclopedia of Ancient Egypt*, Vol. 3, 274–77.

82. G. Robins, "Dress, Undress and the Representation of Fertility and Potency in New Kingdom Egyptian Art," in Kampen, *Sexuality in Ancient Art* (Cambridge: Cambridge University Press, 1996), 25.

generative creation."[83] Color differentiation is thus an important signifier of ideological roles, not simply a natural reflection of actual roles.

Artistic elements, such as male/female color differentiation, are used to form what Shanks has described (in a discussion of stylistic features in Greek art) as "a technology of power" in which "concepts and practices of the self and body, ideas of the powers and limits which are appropriate to both; . . . and aesthetic systems which indicate the appropriateness of action . . . may also work to establish metaphorical links."[84] Color, just as scale and position, is part of a consistent program of representation that reflects the Egyptian ruling elite's view of status and power and re-affirms underlying gender roles.

While male and female are complementary, the male is always the dominant setting. Carved hieroglyphs representing body parts are painted red. The very standardization of this practice has caused even Wilkinson, who provides an otherwise excellent analysis of Egyptian color symbolism in *Symbol and Magic in Egyptian Art*, to characterize this practice as "only natural as is the portrayal of reeds and other plants as green."[85] If it were truly "natural," one would expect yellow (female) hieroglyphs for body parts to be shown as well. This restriction in hieroglyphs emphasizes the dominance of the male principle, which is similarly reflected in Egyptian mythology. Politically, as we have seen, women also played a subordinate role, which is reflected in the artistic repertoire. We have already discussed the instances of "compositional dominance" in sculpture, outlined by Robins, in which position and scale emphasize the importance of the male figure over the female and the limited number of statue types available for depictions of female figures compared to male.

Texts, on the other hand, emphasize the difference between men and women, which is also a necessary component of the correct ordering of the Egyptian universe. When the collective noun *people* is written, the female determinative is often added to the male, indicating that the differentiation is also important to the Egyptians. Both men and women are often addressed in moralistic texts that discuss what the "people" liked or praised.[86] Male/female color differentiation as an artistic device grew out of the political and social conditions of the formative period of Egyptian civilization—the Late Predynastic

83. V. A. Tobin, "Creation Myths," in D. B. Redford, *The Oxford Encyclopedia of Ancient Egypt*, Vol. 1, 469.
84. M. Shanks, *Art and the Early Greek State: An Interpretive Archaeology* (Cambridge: Cambridge University Press, 1999), 211.
85. R. H. Wilkinson, *Symbol and Magic in Egyptian Art*, 110.
86. H. G. Fischer, *Egyptian Women of the Old Kingdom and of the Heracleopolitan Period*, 24, with examples.

period and Early Dynastic periods (3200–2600 BC).[87] During this period most of the features that remained fixtures of Egyptian civilization for millennia were developed. In particular, the concept that was the dominant political and religious manifestation of Egyptian civilization—the rule of a divine pharaoh—was established. In examining this formative period we see the male/female dynamic that underlies the Egyptian world view promoted by and reflected in the use of male/female color differentiation.

Unfortunately, material evidence from the Predynastic period is fragmentary. It is impossible to trace all the steps in the development of the Egyptian political system, but many things can be determined despite the limited evidence. After a period in which rival kingdoms vied for supremacy, Egypt was eventually unified under one ruler. As Michael Rice notes:

> three outstanding achievements must be set to Egypt's account at this time which represent an extraordinary level of creative accomplishment: these are the institution of divine kingship, the concept of the unified political state and the construction of monumental funerary architecture.[88]

The transition to pharaonic rule required an "ideology of justification" that permeated later art and literature. As Wilkinson notes, "The formation of the Egyptian state and the end of the fourth millennium BC crystallized social distinctions in a particularly marked way, placing the king at the apex of the pyramid."[89] Art becomes a vehicle for expressing this ideology. Although some scholars debate whether this was in fact a deliberately controlled artistic program, many factors indicate that it was. Artistic production is placed under the control of the state, and artists are trained in the canonical style. Cult statues, temple decorations for the gods, and images to house pharaoh's spirit throughout the afterlife were used as vehicles to convey his message. It is clear that a deliberate program is being implemented. Even access to materials (hard stone, wood, precious metals, etc.) was under the king's control.[90] Certainly, later Egyptian history contains many examples of artistic change as part of a deliberate ideological program. The most obvious example is the art of the Amarna

---

87. See M. A. Eaverly, "Dark Men, Light Women: Origins of Color as Gender Indicator in Ancient Egypt," in *The World of Women in the Ancient and Classical Near East*, ed. B. Nakhai (London: Cambridge Scholars Publishing, 2008), 1–12.
88. M. Rice, *Egypt's Making: The Origins of Ancient Egypt, 5000–2000 B.C.*, 72.
89. T. A. H. Wilkinson, *Early Dynastic Egypt* (New York: Routledge, 1999), 29.
90. A. Kozloff, "Sculpture: An Overview," in D. B. Redford, *The Oxford Encyclopedia of Ancient Egypt*, Vol. 3, 218.

period designed to promote the religious changes implemented by the pharaoh Akhenaten that will be explored further in Chapter 2.

For emerging Egypt, unification came from the south (Upper Egypt) during the Naqada II or Gerzean period (ca. 3500–3200 BC). Tribal chiefdoms merged and were conquered to create the Egyptian state. The major evidence for social structure and artistic production for this formative period comes from graves at the most important sites (Hierakonpolis, Nqada, el-Amra, Mahasna, Abydos, Mattmar, Gerza, and Minshat Abu Omar).[91] The quantity and the quality of grave goods suggest social stratification is in place. Special cemeteries are set aside for the richest individuals.

The first monumental painting in Egypt is produced for a tomb during this period. This painting and figural decoration painted on pottery suggest the beginnings of the custom of "taking symbolic and real events into the next world."[92] Art in the service of the afterlife has become a part of the Egyptian tradition.

What types of imagery are used in this early funerary art? Pottery provides the major source for iconography during this period. However, the color palette (red paint on buff clay) and the motifs are limited. Among the dominant themes are schematically rendered outline figures of boats, human figures, and occasionally landscape. Figure shape rather than color distinguishes men from women. Women are usually shown as broad-hipped figures, nude from the waist up and wearing a long skirt. Men are usually shown with triangular chests, narrow waists, and erect phalluses.[93]

Men and women are shown in a fashion analogous to the pottery depictions in the clay figurine repertoire. These early clay figurines are very simply shaped—arms, legs, torsos, and neck are all formed from long rolls of clay. Their pinched, undetailed faces resemble a bird's beak. The waist is very narrow. The figurines are not differentiated by skin color—all figures are the red color of the fired clay—but by the indication of the genitals for men (the males wear penis sheaths) and breasts and broader hips for women. The women either wear only a skirt or are nude with the separation between the legs indicated only by an indentation.[94]

---

91. Ibid., 218.
92. K. M. Cialowicz, "Pre-dynastic Period," in Redford, *The Oxford Encyclopedia of Ancient Egypt*, Vol. 3, 64.
93. For examples see A. Capel, "Goddesses: Catalogue Entry 53a and b," in A. Capel and G. Markoe, eds., *Mistress of the House, Mistress of Heaven: Women in Ancient Egypt*, 121–22, and G. Robins, *The Art of Ancient Egypt*, Fig. 23.
94. For examples, see W. S. Smith, *Ancient Egypt as Represented in the Museum of Fine Arts* (Boston: T.

Although every grave does not contain figurines, female figurines are much more numerous.[95] The only context provided for these figurines is their funerary provenance and the iconography of the vases—the range of activities that male and female figures are shown performing in the vases' scenes. These scenes are ambiguous and subject to a variety of interpretations. Female figures are always shown as larger than the males. They are usually shown, like the figurines, with raised arms. They are the subject of much scholarly discussion. Proposed identifications include dancers, mourners, fertility figures, or goddesses.[96] The raised arms could certainly support the mourner or dancer identification. Nudity could argue for fertility figures, although recent scholarship suggests that we are often too quick to identify any pre-historic female figure as related to fertility.[97]

The larger size of the female figures is significant, especially given the fact that in the later canon of Egyptian art scale is manipulated to suggest importance. The larger the figure the more important he or she is in a scene. Size is an indicator of status and is thus highly significant. In searching for a high-status female with which to equate these figures, many scholars have identified them as goddesses.[98]

Hassan suggests that the female figures' upraised arms imitate cow horns and thus connect the figures to a cow goddess, a precursor of the many cow-aspect goddesses of the later Egyptian pantheon.[99] The raised arms of some of the male figurines, although not in the continuous curve exhibited by the females, might be an echo of this.[100] The fact that there are also figures in the same burials that have stump-shaped arms suggests that the upraised arms are not generic and therefore must have been invested with meaning.[101]

O. Metcalf, 1960), Fig. 4, and J. Malek, *Egypt: 4,000 Years of Art*, 502. Fig. 18 Female Figurine, Brooklyn Museum of Art, N.Y. from a grave at El-Mammariyz, height: 33.8cm, collection fund 07.447.

95. B. S. Lesko, *The Great Goddesses of Egypt* (Norman: University of Oklahoma Press, 1991), 10. B. Midant-Reyes, *The Pre-history of Egypt* (Oxford: Wiley Blackwell, 2000), 176, translation by I. Shaw of 1997 original.

96. B. K. Hartwig, "Painting," in D. B. Redford, *The Oxford Encyclopedia of Ancient Egypt*, Vol. 3, 4–5. B. S. Lesko, *The Great Goddesses of Egypt*, 10–11.

97. On this point see L. Goodison and C. Morris, *Ancient Goddesses: The Myths and the Evidence.*

98. B. S. Lesko, *The Great Goddesses of Egypt*, 10–13.

99. F. Hassan, "Primeval Goddess to Divine King: The Mythogenesis of Power in the Early Egyptian State," in *Studies Dedicated to Michael Allen Hoffman*, ed. R. Friedman and B. Adams (Oxford: Egyptian Studies Publications, 1992), 307–21.

100. For an example, see W. S. Smith, *Ancient Egypt as Represented in the Museum of Fine Arts Boston*, Fig. 4. B. S. Lesko, *The Great Goddesses of Egypt*, 15.

101. For an example, see A. Capel and G. Markoe, eds., *Mistress of the House, Mistress of Heaven: Women in Ancient Egypt*, No. 53, 122.

If the arm imagery is in fact evocative of cow imagery, both male and female figurines could reflect a belief system connected with the cattle-herding structure of Predynastic society in which the female is considered the nurturer and source of life. The not-yet-unified local chiefdoms had a religious pantheon based on goddesses and male ithyphallic gods.[102] Further support for the life-giving aspect of the female goddess comes from a female figurine found at Naqada by Petrie that is decorated with images of flora and fauna, perhaps suggesting that the "goddess" is the source of these benefits.[103] While specific identification based solely on the interpretation of images with no written context is very difficult and fraught with the possibility of error, the above discussion does point out a feature of Predynastic society important to our analysis, namely, that women played an important role, at least in the funerary ideology of the period. Predynastic graves provide one area of possible supporting evidence for a status for women equal to or even more prominent than that of men at this time.

Mortuary analysis of Predynastic gravesites suggests equality in tomb size and wealth of offerings between male and female.[104] There are, however, distinctions in spheres of activity. At Cemetery N7000 at Naga-ed Der, Savage identifies eleven artifact clusters that he associates with social roles. Female burials are associated with all eleven, while male burials are associated with seven. Caution must be used since some roles are only represented by a few burials, but it is noteworthy that these patterns suggest a broader range of *at least symbolic* social roles for women than for men.[105] They indicate a society in which women may be equal to or even more important than men.

This evidence is by no means conclusive. Certainly mortuary evidence has its own pitfalls. Intact cemeteries are rare, and there is much debate over the relationship between roles accorded individuals in death and their actual societal roles since funerary ritual may provide a distorted reality by altering or idealizing societal roles. However, such distortion should be in line with the symbolic fabric of a society. The mortuary patterns discussed above suggest a different status for women before pharaonic unification than that which we

---

102. F. Hassan, "Earliest Goddesses of Egypt: Divine Mothers and Cosmic Bodies," in L. Goodison and C. Morris, eds., *Ancient Goddesses: The Myths and the Evidence*, 101.
103. B. S. Lesko, *The Great Goddesses of Egypt*, Fig. 1, 15–16.
104. S. Savage, "The Status of Women in Pre-Dynastic Egypt as Revealed through Mortuary Analysis," in A. Rautmann, *Reading the Body: Representations and Remains in the Archaeological Record* (Philadelphia: University of Pennsylvania Press, 2000), 77–92.
105. Ibid., 86.

have detailed after unification in which the male is clearly dominant. The fact that male/female color differentiation appears only after unification adds support to the idea that such differentiation is part of the mechanism of enforcing/illustrating the new social order.

For our study, however, the question remains whether the absence of the color convention during this time is indeed a reflection of an "egalitarian" situation, and thus ideologically significant, or is simply a function of a limited color palette. A vital piece of evidence in this discussion is the only monumental painting from this period and indeed the earliest yet found in Egypt. The painting, from Tomb 100 at Hierakonpolis, dates to the Naqada II period (3500–3200 BC).[106] As the only painted tomb in the cemetery, it is clearly marked as elite and offers important evidence of the development of the iconography of rule.

The major scene is a procession of six boats. Subsidiary vignettes that include hunting (a person pointing a spear at animals), combat (a figure tying and smiting captives, a bound figure with a mace suspended above), and control of animals (a figure flanked by animals, penned animals) are shown in other scenes. These are all activities that can be connected with the emerging role of chieftainship.[107] Themes that are staples of later Egyptian art are also present. For example, the boats may represent funerary barques, a component of the funerary imagery that becomes so important in later Egyptian art.[108] A connection with power imagery is also suggested by the fact that boats also appear on ceremonial palettes of the later, Dynastic period. A kiosk on the back of one of the Hierakonpolis boats is similar to one shown in the First Dynasty in a depiction of King Den performing the ritual of kingly renewal—the Heb-Sed race.[109] Other features that are important in later dynastic art include the use of scale as an indicator of status (already noted in the discussion of pottery). For example, a figure shown larger than the other figures may be a leader. The smiting of enemies and the mastery of animals, as well as the use of horizontal registers (although without painted ground lines) as the organizing principle of the scenes, are also schema that appear in later Egyptian art. The figure style of

106. H. Case and J. C. Payne, "Tomb 100: The Decorated Tomb at Hierakonpolis," *Journal of Egyptian Archaeology* 48 (1962): 5–18, Pl. 1. T. A. H. Wilkinson, *Early Dynastic Egypt*, 32–33.

107. B. Midant-Reynes, *The Prehistory of Egypt*, 209–10. B. Adams and K. M. Cialowicz, *Protodynastic Egypt* (Buckinghamshire: Shire Publications, 1997), 36. B. J. Kemp, *Ancient Egypt: Anatomy of a Civilization* (London: Routledge, 1989), 47.

108. B. Midant-Reynes, *The Prehistory of Egypt*, 209.

109. B. Adams and K. M. Cialowicz, *Protodynastic Egypt*, 37, Fig. 44e.

the painting is similar to that of the Gerzean pottery and figurines discussed above. The way in which the human body is drawn and the presence of boats link the painting to the artistic tradition of the period.

More significant for our study is the use of color in a potentially symbolic manner—some of the figures are painted black and others red. I use "potentially symbolic" since, as with Gerzean pottery and figurines, the precise meaning of the scenes is impossible to judge. As noted above, the general theme of the painting seems to be the exercise of authority of some figures over others and also over animals. No specific identification is possible for any of the figures or even for the situations depicted and, in fact, the artist's intention may not have been to show an "actual" event.

Nevertheless, colors are used with some degree of consistency, not to distinguish male from female but rather as if they were meant to depict two distinct groups of people. Several red, white, and green ships carry red passengers and face right. Another ship is painted black, as are its passengers, and sails in the opposite direction. It is not possible to securely identify any of the figures in the painting as female based on the typical artistic conventions for depicting women shown on the pottery of the period. Figures placed above the central red boat are in a position analogous to that of the women on pottery but they are not dressed in a similar fashion—they wear long dresses—and they do not exhibit the typical upraised arm gesture of the women on the pottery. They are painted red.

The colors used in the Hierakonpolis painting could be symbolic of two ethnic groups. In dynastic Egyptian art foreigners are distinguished from Egyptians by their skin color. Nubians are painted black, Asiatics yellow. Thus one possible meaning of the two colors is a "realistic" depiction of skin color. That is, the black figures could represent Nubians. While there is clear archaeological evidence of Nubian connections during this period in the form of non-figural pottery characteristic of Nubian Group A,[110] the total scene does not support an identification of "foreign invasion." Although early scholarship attempted to identify some of the ships as foreign, especially Mesopotamian, more recent work has shown that all are types common to Egypt.[111] Based on analysis of the relationships of figures in the scenes and their activities, Case and Payne sug-

110. K. M. Cialowicz, "Pre-Dynastic Period," in D. Redford, *The Oxford Encyclopedia of Ancient Egypt*, Vol. 3, 64.
111. B. Adams and K. M. Cialowicz, *Protodynastic Egypt*, 36.

gest that they are in fact rival political or ethnic groups.[112] Yet no group is seen as the victim or victor in every vignette. A black figure is shown as a conqueror smiting a red person with a mace, while another black figure is shown being speared. A red figure juxtaposed between two lions is shown in the "master of beasts" pose, which—at least in later times—is associated with heroes.[113] A more subtle color use, one that is an important component of color differentiation in pharaonic times, may be at work here, namely, the use of alternating colors to show duality and, by extension, balance between two distinct elements.

The true emphasis, as Case and Payne suggest, is on the restoration of harmony symbolized by the presence of alternating black and red antelopes in the center of the wall and pairs of black and red antelopes elsewhere in the painting.[114] The Hierakonpolis painting would represent a statement of balance. Kemp also sees the painting as a forerunner of later pharaonic symbolism, in which the maintenance of order and balance in the face of the forces of chaos becomes very important.[115] Pharaoh assumes the role of guarantor of harmony. As we have seen, balanced dualities play a major role in later Egyptian art and thought, especially as regards male/female color differentiation. Thus in the Predynastic period many of the motifs that will be mainstays of Egyptian iconography are developed. While symbolic color is one of these features, male/female color differentiation is not. Color differentiation may be absent because the social structure, at least as far as we can read it from mortuary evidence (pottery as well as tombs), suggests a relative equality between men and women. The role of pharaoh, with its consequent emphasis on the dominance of the male principle, has not yet been established. The ideology of the afterlife that supports a role of woman as catalyst has not yet been developed.

A shift away from parity begins to occur as political consolidation under a central male authority begins. The catalyst for change from egality appears to be the consolidation of Egypt under a central dynastic authority. Silverblatt has shown that a shift in the status of women is often a product of state formation.[116] Lerner connects this shift to the Neolithic period and the development

112. H. Case and J. C. Payne, "Tomb 100: The Decorated Tomb at Hierakonpolis," *Journal of Egyptian Archaeology* 48 (1962): 5–18.

113. On this point see B. Adams and K. M. Cialowicz, *Protodynastic Egypt*, 36.

114. H. Case and C. K. Payne, "Tomb 100: The Decorated Tomb at Hierakonpolis," 17.

115. B. J. Kemp, *Ancient Egypt: Anatomy of a Civilization*, 46.

116. I. Silverblatt, "Women in States," *Annual Review of Anthropology* 17 (1988): 427–60.

of agriculture,[117] but again the mortuary evidence indicates that the shift occurs later, during the late Predynastic and Archaic periods, coinciding with the consolidation of pharaonic power.

The specific nature of whatever state is formed determines the ideology behind the diminution of women's status and in particular the way in which women are represented. In Egypt the state emphasizes pharaonic rule. The emergence of pharaonic rule elevates the male pharaoh as a superior force that is both overseer and guarantor of balance. This ideology of rule is manifest in a new religious framework. As Hassan observes, the unification "brought about a dramatic change in ideology, legitimating the role of a national king who incorporated and assimilated earlier deities within a cosmogenic myth that placed him as the descendant and legitimate inheritor of the throne. The change signaled a shift in the role of female deities to a supporting character."[118] The pharaoh—and consequently the male principle—is not only a political force but is also the divine guarantor of the safety and continuity of Egypt. Pharaoh embodies male and female divinities. The king becomes a "manifestation" of the male god Horus, but he also bears titles connected with the "Two Ladies," the goddesses of Lower and Upper Egypt, and with Hathor, the cow goddess. Goddesses "gave birth to kings, nursed and protected them, defended them against their mortal enemies in the underworld and ensured the integrity of their bodies and their health."[119] The recognition of the female principle also finds acknowledgment in the human sphere through the queens of Egypt.[120] While queens formed a female counterpart to the pharaoh, they were not equal in political power and derived what power they had from their association with the male pharaoh. A female ruler—the king's mother Mer-Neith—is attested to during the First Dynasty, but she serves as regent for King Den. Although she has a full mortuary complex at Abydos, her name is not written in the serekh, a designation reserved for pharaohs. Her inscriptions are not prominent outside Abydos, suggesting that most documents carried the king's name.[121]

Art plays a major role in promulgating this world view, especially the concept of pharaonic rule. The ideology of kingship is shown in such early Dynas-

---

117. G. Lerner, *The Creation of Patriarchy* (Oxford: Oxford University Press, 1986), 154.

118. F. Hassan, "Earliest Goddesses of Egypt: Divine Mothers and Cosmic Bodies," in L. Goodison and C. Morris, eds., *Ancient Goddesses: The Myths and the Evidence*, 101.

119. Ibid., 109.

120. L. Troy, *Patterns of Queenship in Ancient Egyptian Myth and History* (Upsala: Acta Universitatis Upsaliensis, 1986), 7–9. See also G. Robins, *Women in Ancient Egypt*, 42.

121. T. A. H. Wilkinson, *Early Dynastic Egypt*, 74–75. A. Capel and G. Markoe, eds., *Mistress of the House, Mistress of Heaven: Women in Ancient Egypt*, 25–30.

tic monuments as the Narmer Palette.[122] One side of the carved slate palette is divided into three registers. The king, much larger than his attendants, wears the Red Crown of Lower Egypt and strides toward decapitated enemies. In the second register men control two entwined long-necked beasts. In the lowest register a bull is trampling a man lying outside a walled enclosure. On the two registers of the other side, pharaoh smites an enemy while a small attendant and the Horus falcon observe. In the lower register beneath the king's feet lie two enemies. All of these images stress the power of the pharaoh over his enemies, his control over Upper and Lower Egypt, and the establishment of unity. While there is debate over whether Narmer actually held the hegemony expressed in this monument, the message is clear.[123] Elements such as the smiting pose will persist throughout Egyptian history as icons of pharaoh's power.

By the Fourth Dynasty there is a codification and stabilization of kingly power and its iconography. Pharaonic rule brought with it a variety of ideological changes emphasizing the dominant male role of the national leader. The result is clearly seen in governmental structure. With several notable exceptions (which will be discussed later in this chapter), the role of pharaoh is reserved for men. The supporting bureaucracy of scribes and government officials is restricted to males. The artistic patterns that support this world view and that will last for millennia are now firmly in place. Among these is the use of male/female color differentiation, the earliest examples of which belong to this period.

The fact that men dominate the government, however, does not mean that women are kept in seclusion. Numerous studies have shown that Egyptian women's lives were not as narrowly constricted as were the lives of women in other parts of the Ancient World. There are clear indications that Egyptian women did have many legal rights not available to their ancient Mediterranean counterparts. Egyptian women could, for example, own property and conduct business. Legally they had rights equal to those of men.[124] Egyptian women held titles referring to roles in temple ritual and positions at court, indicating that their sphere of activity was not confined to the home.[125] Textual evidence shows that women were vital to one of the most important industries in Egypt,

---

122. Cairo, Egyptian Museum from Hierakonpolis. G. Robins, *The Art of Ancient Egypt*, Fig. 25.

123. For a discussion of opinions, see S. Vinson, "Narmer," in D. B. Redford, *The Oxford Encyclopedia of Ancient Egypt*, Vol. 2, 494–95.

124. On this point see G. Robins, *Reflections of Women in the New Kingdom: Ancient Egyptian Art from the New Kingdom* (Atlanta: Emory University, 1995), 4.

125. Ibid., 14, and G. Robins, "Women," in Redford, *The Oxford Encyclopedia of Ancient Egypt*, Vol. 3, 512.

fabric weaving, even holding the office of supervisor.[126] Elite women were also involved in supervising lower-class women in large-scale operations such as baking, brewing, and winnowing.

In addition to women's legal status and ability to conduct business affairs in their own right, these activities indicate that their lives were not sequestered. It is an oversimplification to say that women in Egyptian art are shown as pale because they are kept indoors. Basing such a judgment on the artistic repertoire alone is assuming that those depictions provide photographically realistic images of Egyptian life, and that is obviously not the case. The artistic repertoire does not reflect the variety of roles and occupations available to women. Women's supervisory and temple activities are very seldom shown. The offices they held are seldom acknowledged in art. While statues of men are labeled with titles indicating the offices they hold, women are usually identified simply as wives. From the Middle Kingdom onward women were given the title "Mistress of the House."[127] This designation suggests that women's sphere of activity was primarily domestic, a contrast with the political offices held by men. However, this epithet implies relative domains between men and women rather than any sequestering of women within the home. Color could thus be a way to indicate these separate spheres of activity rather than any actual harem-like seclusion for women.

While women did not hold governmental offices, there was, as described above, one politically important role open to them, namely, that of queen.[128] In Dynastic Egypt, royal succession normally passed from father to son. Thus kings needed royal women to produce their heirs. In addition to their reproductive duties, "King's mothers" and the king's principal wife played a ritual role. As the bearers of divine queenship, they complemented the divine aspect of kingship.

While the pharaoh was a "male" office—pharaoh was the representative of the god Horus on earth—from the earliest period of pharaonic rule there was provision for a woman to rule in exceptional circumstances, usually as regent

---

126. C. H. Roehrig, "Women's Work: Some Occupations of Nonroyal Women as Depicted in Ancient Egyptian Art," in A. Capel and G. Markoe, eds., *Mistress of the House, Mistress of Heaven: Women in Ancient Egypt*, 19–24.

127. On this title see A. Capel and G. Markoe, eds., *Mistress of the House, Mistress of Heaven: Women in Ancient Egypt*, passim.

128. The standard work on queens is L. Troy, *Patterns of Queenship in Ancient Egyptian Myth and History*. See also G. Robins, "Gender Roles," in Redford, *The Oxford Encyclopedia of Ancient Egypt*, Vol. 2, 12–16; Z. Hawass, *Silent Images: Women in Pharaonic Egypt* (New York: America University in Cairo Press, 1999), 26–35; and J. Tydesley, *Chronicles of the Queens of Egypt*.

for a son too young to assume the throne. The documentation is scanty, but three examples are preserved from the Old Kingdom. The earliest was Neith-Hotep who ruled for Djer, possibly her nephew. Her role was that of regent, not pharaoh. Later women who served as regents were usually identified with the title of "King's Mother." The first documented holder of this title is Mer-Neith in the Mid First Dynasty. Her tomb is preserved but there are no representations of her.[129] The fact that the tomb is identified by inscription as hers rather than as that of a husband or male relative indicates her high status. Owning a tomb is generally a male prerogative. Elite women are usually buried in their husband's funerary chapels and do not have stand-alone funerary complexes.[130] Yet Mer-Neith did not carry the full nomenclature of a pharaoh. These women were not regarded as rulers in their own right, although they exercised considerable power.[131]

There is, however, one possible Old Kingdom example of a woman who ruled as pharaoh rather than regent. Nitokret is only attested to from literary sources much later than her presumed reign at the end of the Sixth Dynasty, and her existence has been questioned. If she did indeed rule, the fact that she was pharaoh at the *end* of a dynasty suggests that an exception may have been made because there was no male successor available. Bloodlines would have taken precedence over gender. This again seems to be the case at the end of the Twelfth Dynasty when another female pharaoh, Sobekneferu, is attested to. Evidence for both of these women is fragmentary.[132] It is clear from these examples that a female ruler was a very rare occurrence in ancient Egypt. Pharaoh was primarily a male role, and in the correct ordering of the universe political power belonged to the male sphere. There is thus a division of activity between female and male roles. Women did not stay within the house, but their ideal role was one in which they were in charge of domestic activities.

Hieroglyphic writing provides a flexible medium for the transmission of written messages. Individual hieroglyphic characters can depict actual objects,

---

129. On these women see B. Bryan, "In Woman Good and Bad Fortune Are on Earth: Status and Roles of Women in Egyptian Culture," in A. Capel and G. Markoe, eds., *Mistress of the House, Mistress of Heaven: Women in Ancient Egypt*, 28–29.

130. H. G. Fischer, *Egyptian Women of the Old Kingdom and of the Heracleopolitan Period*, 2–9.

131. A. M. Roth, "Models of Authority: Hatshepsut's Predecessors in Power," in *Hatshepsut from Queen to Pharaoh*, ed. C. H. Roehrig (New York: Metropolitan Museum of Art, 2005).

132. B. Bryan, "In Woman Good and Bad Fortune Are on Earth: Status and Roles of Women in Egyptian Culture," in A. Capel and G. Markoe, eds., *Mistress of the House, Mistress of Heaven: Women in Ancient Egypt*, 29; A. M. Roth, "Models of Authority: Hatshepsut's Predecessors in Power," in C. H. Roehrig, ed., *Hatshepsut from Queen to Pharaoh*, 7.

can be used in a metaphorical manner to suggest another object, or can be combined to express a concept. They can have a variety of meanings within the Egyptian system. Within this framework male/female color differentiation functions as a metaphorical statement—the light color chosen for women's skin indicates a virtual sequestering. By painting women white or yellow, Egyptian artists define an ideal interior realm for women, one that marks an elite woman whether she is actually inside or not. Color is part of the stylistic repertoire, the decorum that asserts roles for male and female in accordance with the correct ordering of the universe. Male/female color differentiation is but one aspect of the artistic canon that supports the male-centered ideology that is introduced by pharaonic rule. It marks the distinct spheres of male/female activity but also serves to show that they are complementary. The union of opposites represented by the two colors emphasizes the completion created by joining male and female. This combination functions just as the joining of two hieroglyphic symbols to create a concept broader than simply the presence of its individual components. Color differentiation works within the symbolic artistic color system established by the Egyptians not only to suggest difference but also to suggest that both male and female are vital for the correct ordering of the universe. The dominance of the male principle is also emphasized in such practices as the use of dark skin as the default setting for hieroglyphs indicating body parts and in the greater fluidity with which color can be used to depict male divinities. The indoor/outdoor explanation for the difference in skin tone between men and women in Egyptian art has tended to simplify what was a much more complex process.

Symbolism is thus a vital part of color use in Egypt. Visual cues are important in interpreting color in Egypt because color denotes the category to which each object belongs. The Egyptian interest in categories reflects a world view that emphasized the unchanging aspects of objects rather than their transitory states. As we have seen, certain symbolic aspects of male/female color differentiation seem to override any "natural," that is, transitory, considerations. Regardless of the activity women are engaged in they are painted the traditional color. This symbolic use of color indicates the emphasis on permanence typical of Egyptian painting and sculpture. In light of the artistic and political features discussed above, it does not seem likely that skin color was necessarily a "realistic" feature. We have already seen that women's spheres of activity were by no means confined to the indoors. Pale skin is not necessarily a reflection of lack of sun exposure brought on by seclusion. It reflects symbolic rather than actual roles.

CHAPTER 2

Egypt

The Exception That Proves the Rule— Hatshepsut and Akhenaten

As we have seen in Chapter 1, male/female color differentiation supports an ideology established and promoted by pharaonic rule in which male and female are complementary opposites. Male/female color differentiation is the visual manifestation of this ideal. However, significant changes to this representational system occur during the reigns of two New Kingdom pharaohs: Hatshepsut and Akhenaten. These two periods of profound difference emphasize the close connection between color as gender indicator and pharaonic ideology; they are in a sense "the exception that proves the rule." Each of these pharaohs alters the standard ideology, although for different purposes. Male/female color differentiation plays an important part in articulating the changes presented during each of their reigns.

The first alteration in the established Egyptian artistic tradition is the twenty-year rule of the *female* pharaoh Hatshepsut. During her reign artists wrestled with the portrayal of a female occupant of an office whose symbolism and iconography are traditionally gendered male. The second alteration in standard procedure is the religious revolution of the pharaoh Akhenaten. Akhenaten, originally Amenhotep IV, replaces the traditional pantheon of gods with worship of the sun god, the Aten. His "revolution" alters not only the structure of Egyptian religion but also fundamental beliefs about the nature of the universe and the afterlife. Hatshepsut modifies the convention to accommodate the fact that although she is pharaoh she is also a woman. Akhenaten eliminates the color distinction between men and women as part of his radical re-ordering of the Egyptian pantheon. During Hatshepsut's reign dark color becomes appropriate for Hatshepsut, but not necessarily for every woman.

During Akhenaten's reign male and female are painted the same dark color. The fact that both of these "crisis" points in Egyptian society involve a change in the use of male/female color differentiation further strengthens my contention that this artistic feature does not simply represent a difference in sun exposure between men and women, but instead reflects deeper underlying societal values established and promoted by pharaoh.

We would expect that if color differentiation were simply "conventional" it would be an unchanging "given" of Egyptian art. Instead, the change in monuments produced during the reign of each of these pharaohs clearly shows that the use of color as gender indicator is highly symbolic. When "normalcy" (i.e., standard practice) is restored after each of their reigns, male/female color differentiation also returns to its traditional and standard form—dark men, light women. These two critical periods are fundamental for our understanding of the role of male/female color differentiation within the Egyptian artistic tradition. The changes instigated by each of these pharaohs spotlight just how closely male/female color differentiation connects to underlying ideology.

Hatshepsut's reign poses the intriguing question of what happens to royal iconography when the role of pharaoh, a position traditionally gendered male and an icon of male power, is assumed by a woman. In Chapter 1, I showed that the development of pharaonic rule was accompanied by an emphasis on the male principle in the religious and artistic spheres. As part of this, pharaoh was clearly identified as a male and was the male god Horus's earthly manifestation. Hatshepsut, a woman who claims the title of pharaoh, must contend with this male-centered ideology to maintain her position as head of the Egyptian state. She is not the first woman to rule Egypt, but hers is the longest and most clearly documented reign, and she is one of only two women who assumed the title of pharaoh. To understand further the uniqueness of her position, we need to examine the relatively rare examples of women rulers in Egypt. As I have said, women usually served as regent for a male relative who was too young to assume the throne, not as rulers in their own right. Each female ruler was usually identified with the title "King's Mother." Nitokret, the one Old Kingdom example of a woman who ruled as pharaoh rather than regent, is only attested to from literary sources much later than her presumed reign and her existence has been questioned.[1]

1. B. Bryan, "In Woman Good and Bad Fortune are on Earth: Status and Roles of Women in Egyptian Culture," in *Mistress of the House, Mistress of Heaven: Women in Ancient Egypt*, ed. A. Capel and G. Markoe (New York: Hudson Hills Press, 1996), 29; A. M. Roth, "Models of Authority: Hatshepsut's

During the Middle Kingdom we have the first clearly documented example of a female pharaoh. Sobeknefru[2] was the daughter of the Twelfth Dynasty King Amenemhat III. Rather than serving as regent, she held the complete royal titulary associated with pharaoh. She is called "The Horus, She Who Is Beloved of Ra, She of the Two Ladies, Powerful Daughter, Mistress of the Two Lands, the Golden Falcon, Enduring of Appearances, the King of Upper and Lower Egypt, Sobekkar, The Daughter of Ra Sobeknefru."[3] These titles make it clear that she is both pharaoh and female. The fact that she is a woman is also clearly indicated in the fragmentary sculptural depictions of her. The best preserved is a statue in the Louvre, although all that remains of the original is a portion of the torso from the base of the neck to just above the thighs and attached arm fragments.[4] The statue is frontal. The traces of the arms show that she held them at her sides, indicating that she was standing rather than seated. There are no traces of paint, but enough of the statue remains to show that her body is female. Breasts are clearly indicated beneath the sheath she wears. However, she also wears a male kilt over the dress, and the lappets of the *nemes*, the traditional pharaonic—and thus male—headdress, are clearly shown falling onto her shoulders just above her breasts. Her statue thus combines her biological gender with the symbols of the traditionally male role of pharaoh. Since no paint is preserved we cannot tell whether her skin was depicted with the traditional reddish-brown paint used to indicate males or the yellow used for females.

Sobeknefru's reign was clearly an unusual circumstance. Millennia had passed without a female pharaoh. A male assuming the male role was the norm. A female pharoah was not the preferred situation. The combination of female secondary sexual characteristics and male and female costume shown in her statue is the artist's solution to the problem of a female occupant of a male office. Because her reign was so atypical, she needed to bolster her legitimacy. An inscription on a red granite column promotes the fact that her reign is supported by her (male) predecessor. On this column her father's Horus name of-

Predecessors in Power," in *Hatshepsut from Queen to Pharaoh*, ed. C. Roehrig (New York: Metropolitan Museum of Art, 2005), 7.

2. R. A. Gillam, "Sobekneferu," in *The Oxford Encyclopedia of Ancient Egypt*, Vol. 3, ed. D. Redford (Oxford: Oxford University Press, 2001), 301.
3. B. Bryan, "In Woman Good and Bad Fortune are on Earth: Status and Roles of Women in Egyptian Culture," in A. Capel and G. Markoe, eds., *Mistress of the House, Mistress of Heaven: Women in Ancient Egypt*, 29.
4. Louvre E 27135. Ibid., 30, Fig. 7.

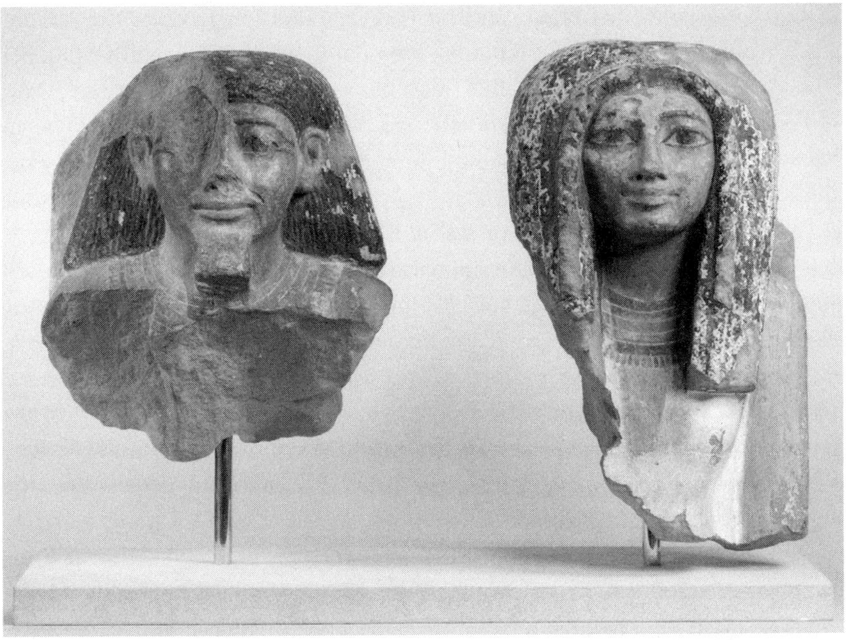

Fig. 7. Pair of male and female busts. Egyptian; Thebes probably. New Kingdom, reign of Thutmose I-Thutmose III, ca. 1504–1425 BC. Sandstone, paint. Male bust: H. 14 1/8 in (35.8 cm); w. 11 15/16 in (30.3 cm); d. 8 3/4 in (22.2 cm); Female bust: H. 17 1/16 in (43.4 cm); w. 10 1/16 in (25.5 cm); d. 9 in (22.8 cm). Left: Male bust (13.182.1a); right: Female bust (13.182.1b). (Rogers Fund, 1913 [13.182.1a, b]. The Metropolitan Museum of Art, NY, U.S.A. Image © The Metropolitan Museum of Art/Art Resource, NY.)

fers the sign of life and stability to her Horus name. This transfer indicates that it was the male pharaoh, her father, who desired that she rule.[5] Sobeknefru navigates the iconographically tricky situation of being a woman in a male role by adding male costume to her statuary and linking her legitimacy to a traditional male figure. The scanty preservation of her monuments precludes discovering how she adapted or worked within the traditional male/female skin color scheme shown in Figure 7.

Hatshepsut is the only other well-documented case of a female pharaoh.

5. I. Harari, "Nature de la stele de donation de function du roi Ahmosis à la reine Ahmês Nefertari," *ASAE* 56 (1959): 139–201; Pl. 1.

Unlike Sobeknefru, her reign was long (twenty years compared to four). Consequently, we should have much more material to work with in examining her iconography and interpreting the forces that shaped her reign. However, most of her monuments were either defaced or destroyed by her successor. Questions remain about why she assumed the throne in the first place and why her successor attacked her monuments nearly two decades after her death. Possible reasons for this "*damnatio memoriae*" will be discussed later in this chapter.

Some facts are clear. Hatshepsut was the daughter of pharaoh Thutmose I and his wife Ahmose and was herself the wife of her half brother who became pharaoh Thutmose II. The product of their marriage was a daughter. During this time Hatshepsut's inscriptions stressed her status as "God's Wife of Amen," a traditional title for queens, most securely attested to for the first half of the Eighteenth Dynasty.[6] Thutmose II died prematurely, leaving behind a young son by a woman named Isis. Hatshepsut began her rule as regent for that son, who was the chosen successor as pharaoh and was named Thutmose III. As regent, she continued to emphasize her title as "God's Wife of Amen." At some point between the second and seventh year of this co-rule Hatshepsut assumed full power and was crowned pharaoh. Exactly when this coronation occurred is unclear, since she always dates her reign to the beginning of the regency.[7]

Various theories have been proposed as to why she felt it necessary to take on the role of pharaoh rather than continuing as regent. Scholarly views have shifted from twentieth-century descriptions of a scheming power-hungry femme fatale to more recent assessments that suggest that the move was necessary to hold the throne for Thutmose III.[8] Regardless of motive, Hatshepsut did assume the throne as pharaoh and ruled for twenty years. As we have seen, a female in the iconically male role was the exception, never the rule. Hatshepsut thus had to create an ideology and iconography that would legitimize her position. The length of her reign indicates that she was able to do this successfully.

We have seen that Sobeknefru, the only other clearly documented female pharaoh, combined male and female elements in her statuary. She provided a precedent for Hatshepsut that differs from that of the Queen mothers, the fe-

---

6. See L. Troy, *Patterns of Queenship in Ancient Egyptian Myth and History* (Upsala: Acta Universitatis Upsaliensis, 1986), 141; G. Robins, *Women in Ancient Egypt* (London, 1993), 42.

7. A. M. Roth, "Models of Authority: Hatshepsut's Predecessors in Power," in C. H. Roehrig, ed., *Hatshepsut from Queen to Pharaoh*, 12.

8. C. Keller, "Hatshepsut's Reputation in History," in C. H. Roehrig, *Hatshepsut from Queen to Pharaoh*, 294–97; A. M. Roth, "Models of Authority: Hatshepsut's Predecessors in Power," in C. H. Roehrig, *Hatshepsut from Queen to Pharaoh*, 12.

male regents, whose imagery was always gendered female. While she is acting as official regent, Hatshepsut's iconography shifts from purely female depictions to a mixture of male and female elements. However, after her accession to the throne, male imagery predominates.

The early female imagery is represented by several reliefs, none of which, unfortunately, has preserved paint. In a graffito from Aswan, Hatshepsut is dressed in the clothing of a queen, holding the insignia of the God's Wife of Amun.[9] In a relief from the Temple of Semna in Nubia, Thutmose II is shown as king. Hatshepsut stands beside him, wearing a traditional long female dress and labeled with the titles of a queen.[10] Thus, in both of these depictions she is queen and not pharaoh.

As mentioned above, the exact date of her coronation as pharaoh is debated. One piece of evidence that suggests an early step toward complete rule is her use of a new prenomen, essentially a coronation name: Maatkare. This is written inside a cartouche, an enclosure usually reserved for pharaoh's names. Hatshepsut, however, is still portrayed in female costume and accompanied by the title of God's Wife, typically used for a queen in images associated with this name.[11] At this stage she combines a pharaonic title with a queenly image. In later works she moves away from the queenly image and combines a female body and dress with pharaonic (male) power symbols. In a quartzite relief (again the paint is not preserved) from a chapel at Karnak she wears a typical long, tight-fitting female gown, together with the pharaonic plumed crown with ram's horn. The inscriptions in front of her cartouches label her "King of Upper and Lower Egypt" and "Mistress of Ritual."[12] Both image and titles combine male and female elements. The lack of preserved paint on these early images leaves us unable to answer the question of which gender she identified with according to the color convention.

However, a series of colossal statues from her funerary complex at Deir el-

9. L. Habachi, "Two Graffitti at Sehēl from the Reign of Queen Hatshepsut," *Journal of Near Eastern Studies*, 16 (April 1957): 92–96; F. Dorman, "Hatshepsut: Princess to Queen to Co-Ruler," in C. H. Roehrig, ed., *Hatshepsut from Queen to Pharaoh*, 88.

10. R. A. Caminos, *Semna-Kumma, Vol. 1: The Temple of Semma, Archaeological Survey of Egypt, Thirty-seventh Memoir* (London: Egypt Exploration Society, 1988), 42; F. Dorman (2005), "Hatshepsut: Princess to Queen to Co-Ruler," in C. H. Roehrig, ed., *Hatshepsut from Queen to Pharaoh*, 88.

11. G. Robins, "The Names of Hatshepsut as King," *Journal of Egyptian Archaeology* 85 (1999): 109–12; A. H. Gardiner, T. E. Peet, and J. Černý, eds., *The Inscriptions of Sinai* (Oxford: Oxford: Egypt Exploration Society, 1952–55), No. 1777, Pl. LVI.

12. H. Chevrier, "Rapport sur les travaux de Karnak (1933–34)," *Annales du Service des Antiquités de l'Égypte*, 34 (March–May 1926): 172, Pl. IV; F. Dorman, "Hatshepsut: Princess to Queen to Co-Ruler," in C. H. Roehrig, ed., *Hatshepsut from Queen to Pharaoh*, Fig. 38.

Bahri provides important evidence for her color/gender choices. Her mortuary temple is decorated with three series of engaged limestone statues. These statues are usually identified as images of her as Osiris, thus presenting her in the guise of a deceased ruler, a typical depiction for a pharaonic mortuary temple.[13] Arnold sees the statues simply as "symbols of eternal, divine, kingship." Her statues are unparalleled in that she is presented as grasping an unprecedented combination of pharaonic implements, two flails in the left hand and a crook and scepter in the right,[14] almost a case of "overkill" with pharaonic (male) symbols. She wears a garment composed of a Sedfestival (jubilee) cloak, symbolic of the ritual renewal festival that pharaohs underwent during their reigns. She also wears a tightly wrapped mummiform sheath, indicating the funerary nature of the monument.

The statues are found at different locations within the complex. Four are in the sanctuary itself. Ten are attributed to the rear niches of the upper terrace. Twenty-six appear across the front of the upper terrace portico. According to the stylistic chronology established by Tefnin, each of the above groupings dates to a different period during Hatshepsut's reign. The four from the inner temple complex comprise the earliest group.[15] These statues are particularly important to our study since the paint is preserved. Hatshepsut is shown with the yellow flesh color usually reserved for women, as seen in Figure 8. All of the other statues from the mortuary temple are painted with dark brown paint, the traditional male color (Figure 9). If Tefnin's chronology is correct, the yellow statues belong to the earliest phase of her rule. Their yellow skin color would be an appropriate expression of Hatshepsut's early iconography in which she, like Sobeknefru before her, combines male power imagery with female physical characteristics and costume.

A different approach, this time combining male flesh color with female physical characteristics, occurs in a relief from her Hathor temple, also at Deir el-Bahri. In this scene, Hatshepsut, painted the typical brown male color but with (damaged, but still visible) breasts, is being nursed by the goddess Hathor (depicted as a cow). The image emphasizes the pharaoh's connection to the goddess who literally nourishes Hatshepsut.[16] In the early Osiride statues from

13. Although they are generally identified as Osirides. D. Arnold, "The Temple of Hatshepsut at Deir el-Bahri," in C. H. Roehrig, ed., *Hatshepsut from Queen to Pharaoh*, 138.

14. C. Keller, "The Statuary of Hatshepsut," in C. H. Roehrig, ed., *Hatshepsut from Queen to Pharaoh*, 160.

15. R. Tefnin, *La statuaire d'Hatshepsout: Portrait royal et politique sous la 18e Dynastie* (Brussels: Fondation Egyptologique Reine, 1997), 38–40.

16. A. M. Roth, "Erasing a Reign," in C. H. Roehrig, ed., *Hatshepsut from Queen to Pharaoh*, Fig. 102; P.

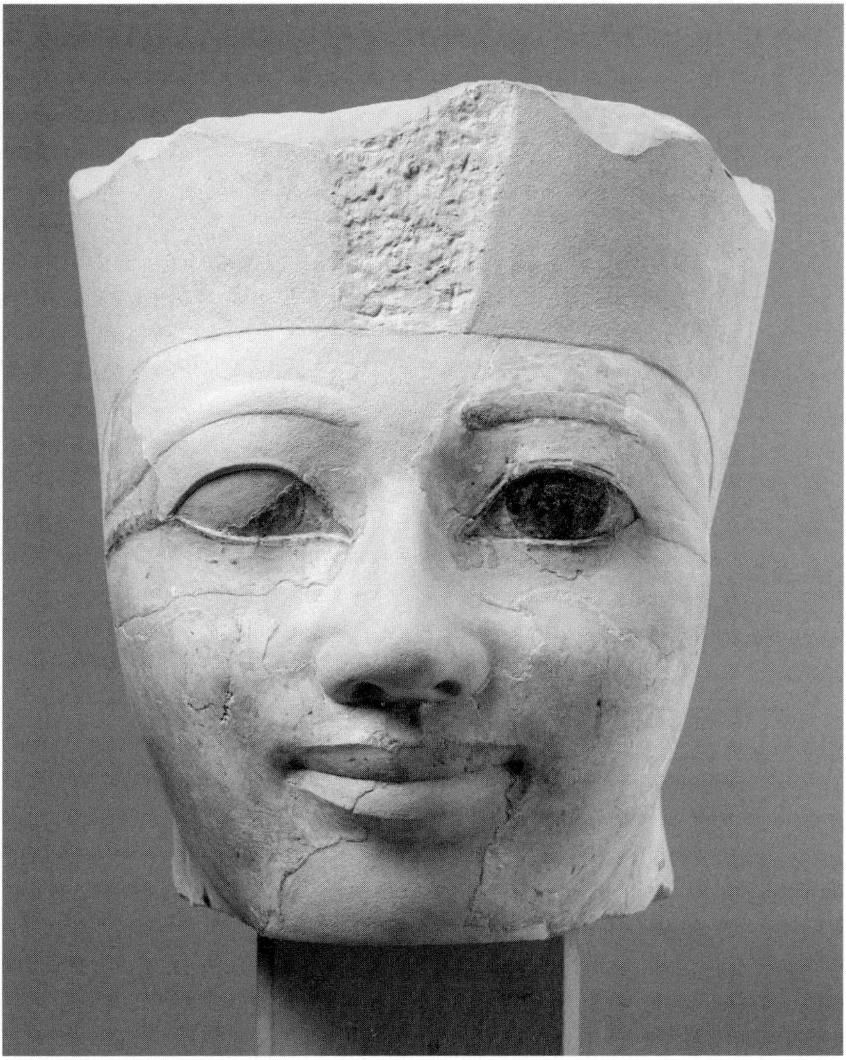

Fig. 8. Head of an osiride statue of Hatshepsut. Egyptian; Thebes, Deir el-Bahri. New Kingdom, Joint reign of Hatshepsut and Thutmose III, ca. 1473–1458 BC. Limestone, paint, H. 8 11/16 in (22 cm). (Rogers Fund, 1931 [31.3.154]. The Metropolitan Museum of Art, New York, NY, U.S.A. Image © The Metropolitan Museum of Art/Art Resource, NY.)

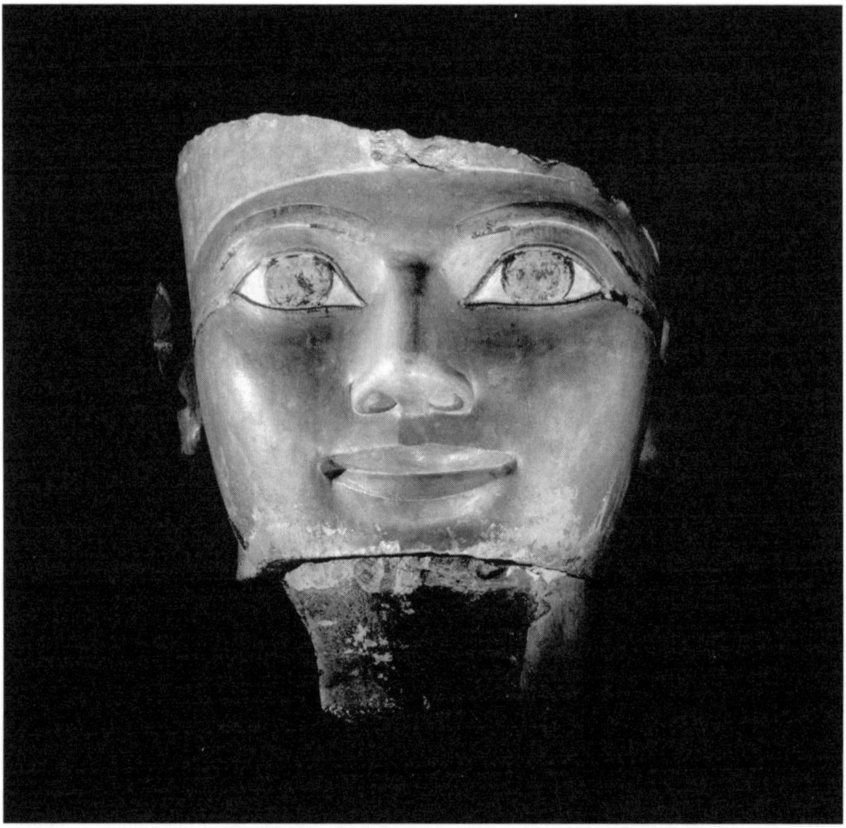

Fig. 9. Head of Hatshepsut. Fragment of a statue from the queen's temple at Deir el-Bahari representing Hatshepsut in the form of Osiris. Eighteenth Dynasty (1490–1470 BC). (Egyptian Museum, Cairo, Egypt. Photo Credit: Werner Forman/Art Resource NY.)

Deir el-Bahri and in this relief, skin color is being used in a manner contrary to some of the other visual cues presented in the sculpture. The skin of the otherwise male Osiride statue is painted the typical female color, while in the relief figure, Hatshepsut, marked as female by the presence of breasts, is painted the usual brown color of male flesh. In both instances male/female color differentiation is a major component of Hatshepsut's endeavor to combine her "two genders"—her biological femaleness and her male iconic role as pharaoh.

Gilbert, "Les sens des portraits intacts de Hatshepsout à Deir el-Bhari," *Chronique d'Egypte*, No. 56 (1953), 219–22.

Some scholars have suggested that Hatshepsut was attempting to create a new conception of pharaoh as an androgynous being embodying male and female. Yet Hatshepsut's images are, in fact, not truly androgynous. The gender markers are confined to skin color and regalia. Secondary sexual characteristics are never combined in these statues. The bodies are either male or female.[17] Hatshepsut is never shown with male genitalia. Instead of combining male and female, she may be attempting to "feminize" the role of pharaoh or at least to normalize, that is, make more palatable and familiar, the concept of a female pharaoh by working within the traditional male/female iconographic framework previously established in Egyptian art through such devices as male/female color differentiation. To this end she also sometimes uses the feminine grammatical form of pharaonic titulary for images of Thutmose III and retroactively applies these feminized forms to Thutmose I and II.[18] This suggests that she may be implying that the titles themselves, and hence the role of pharaoh, need not be confined to males. Her use of feminine terminology to refer to males "universalizes" the title *pharaoh*.

Her later statues, however, indicate that legitimizing her claim to the throne by expanding the role of pharaoh to include feminine attributes was not a successful strategy. She abandons any attempt at combining features in her later art and adopts a purely male persona. We can see this in the groups of Osiride statues from Deir el-Bahri, dated by Tefnin to the latter part of her reign. They represent the shift to male imagery not only in dress but also in skin color. Rather than the yellow color of the earlier Osiride statues from this same complex, these later figures are painted the dark color usually reserved for males. In addition, she follows the traditional pattern of providing a female counterpart to pharaoh, a queen, by naming her own daughter, Neferure, "God's Wife of Amen," a title Hatshepsut herself had held while regent before she assumed the role of pharaoh.[19]

Hatshepsut's use of skin color in her early "combination" works and in these later strictly male creations clearly emphasizes the symbolic nature of male/female color differentiation. Since she is a woman, a traditional depiction of Hatshepsut should have light-colored flesh. Throughout her reign male/female color differentiation is consistently used in the standard form—dark male/light female—for non-pharaonic images. Elite tomb images of nobles and other im-

---

17. On this point see J. Tydesley, *Hatchepsut* (London: Penguin, 1996), 135–36.
18. A. M. Roth, "Models of Authority: Hatshepsut's Predecessors in Power," in C. H. Roehrig, ed., *Hatshepsut from Queen to Pharaoh*, Note 10.
19. L. Troy, *Patterns of Queenship in Ancient Egyptian Myth and History*, 140.

portant officials use the standard colors. The ideological framework of difference between male and female remains intact. Her own depictions show different strategies devised to adapt to this persistent Egyptian framework. When she switches to the dark male skin color for her images, the change is symbolic not of her own sex but of the gender associated with pharaonic power. The imagery of pharaonic rule has always been predominantly male. A female pharaoh is, as we have said, an oddity.

However, her inscriptions consistently use the feminine grammatical form. This seeming dichotomy is based on several factors. First and foremost is that everyone knew that Hatshepsut was a woman. She had been married to a king and served as regent for a king. She had a daughter. Her previous identity as King's Wife was securely established. Additionally, although the role of the pharaoh in the Egyptian system was gendered male, pharaoh's function within that system meant that Hatshepsut could not deny her biological gender. Because the king provided a vital link between the Egyptian people and the gods, pharaonic images served as magical representations of that link. As Roth states, "Her femininity was an essential part of her identity, and images that showed a fictional, nonexistent man named Hatshepsut would not be effective."[20] Any image had to be labeled with her "correct" and thus female name. Hatshepsut had to maintain simultaneously the male power trappings and her biological gender. Hatshepsut's attempts to "stretch" the definition of kingship to include females might have also been prompted by a desire to secure the succession for her daughter. Neferure takes on the typically kingly duty of making offerings to Hathor in an inscription from Sinai, during Year 11 of Hatshepsut's reign. In this same inscription she is given epithets that are usually reserved for a king.[21]

As I have said, Hatshepsut's attempts to combine male and female imagery early in her reign do not appear to have been successful enough to legitimize her rule, since she switched to male skin color for her images and a totally male appearance. Further evidence for her lack of success with the blended male/female image is suggested by her creation of a "foundation myth" to justify her reign. She apparently needed more ammunition to support her claim to the throne. According to the story illustrated in relief sculpture on the north side of the middle portico of her mortuary temple at Deir el- Bahri, Amun, disguised

20. A. M. Roth, "Models of Authority, Hatshepsut's Predecessors in Power," in C. H. Roehrig, ed., *Hatshepsut from Queen to Pharaoh*, 9.

21. D. B. Redford, *History and Chronology of the Eighteenth Dynasty of Egypt: Seven Studies* (Toronto: University of Toronto Press, 1967), 84–85.

as Hatshepsut's father (Thutmose I), impregnated her mother, Queen Ahmose. Hatshepsut is thus fathered by a god. Such a tale of divine impregnation was a traditional part of the male iconography of pharaonic rule. Every pharaoh was the divine son of Amun-Re. In Hatshepsut's case, however, the reliefs and the accompanying text document Amun's decision to have a *daughter* who will rule Egypt rather than the traditional son. This myth presented her as the divinely designated successor of Thutmose I and the God Amun.[22]

While the text makes it very clear that Hatshepsut was ordained *daughter* of the god, the images of the resulting child show her as a naked *boy*. The message seems to be that although Amun knows that boys/men are the usual occupants of the throne, he fully approves of a woman pharaoh in the person of his daughter Hatshepsut.[23] These scenes clearly indicate that during this later period of her reign Hatshepsut chose to adopt the male physiognomy traditionally associated with power. Paint is not preserved from these reliefs, but one would expect the red-brown male color to be used on these images as they belong to the later period in which only the hieroglyphic inscriptions indicate her female gender.

The fact that she felt it necessary to change her image to one that was completely male suggests that her biological gender did cause a problem for the Egyptians. Male iconography was vital to the concept of pharaoh. Neither clothing, as in the case of her early Osiride statues, nor male skin color, as in the relief of Hatshepsut being nursed by Hathor, was sufficient to alter the traditional concept of pharaoh as male. Combined uses of color were eventually rejected just as were combined forms of costume in favor of completely male images. In this milieu color functions in a highly symbolic way, either indicating Hatshepsut's true gender in an otherwise totally male statue, such as the Osirides from Deir el-Bahri, or establishing her assumed gender in otherwise female images such as the nursing scene from the Hathor temple. In her later sculpture, color supplements the complete fiction of a male pharaoh. Hatshepsut's experimentation with the male/female color convention clearly shows that this use of color had a strong symbolic meaning. Color can convey one gender (female) even while all other clues point to another (male).

Although the number of examples of art from her reign with preserved paint is limited, they do suggest that her experiments with using dark skin color

22. E. Naville, *The Temple of Deir el- Bahri, Part 2* (London: Egypt Exploration Fund, 1896), 15; J. Tydesley, *Hatchepsut*, 103–5.
23. J. Tydesley, *Hatchepsut*, 102.

for females were confined to images of Hatshepsut herself and not others. A wall painting from the upper Anubis chapel of her temple at Deir el-Bahri shows Thutmose I and his mother. He is painted the traditional dark male color and his mother the yellow female color.[24] Another image from Deir el-Bahri presents an intriguing variation on male/female color differentiation. In this relief celebrating Hatshepsut's expedition to the land of Punt, the chieftain of the region and his wife are both painted with the dark color usually reserved for Egyptian male flesh. Each does, however, have distinctive "ethnographic" features. The wife is quite fat with pronounced steopygia, and the chieftain wears a long beard and distinctive costume. Skin color in this case functions as an ethnographic marker of an observable feature. On a deeper level the shared skin color might be an attempt to suggest ethnic "sympathy" between the inhabitants of Punt and the Egyptians by means of skin color.[25] In this case an affinity with the Egyptians would be stressed over gender distinctions.

Hatshepsut's lengthy reign indicates that her strategy of assuming male trappings and physiognomy was successful. However, under her successor and co-ruler Thutmose III, her monuments suffered deliberate attacks designed to erase her image.[26] Scholars debate whether these attacks are because of her identity as a woman or because of other political considerations. Arguing for the former reason is the fact that the monuments of the other woman known to rule as pharaoh in her own right, Sobeknefru, also suffered deliberate destruction.[27] This contrasts with the fate of Queen Mothers who continued to be honored for generations after their deaths. If anger at her gender was one of the reasons for the attacks against her monuments, one might expect that monuments that depicted her as a woman would suffer the most. However, no such pattern can be found among the damaged monuments. Male and female images are defaced or destroyed. However, greater vehemence against her as a woman is shown in the *pattern* of destruction against her inscriptions. Her identifying cartouches are systematically erased. In particular, her nomen—

---

24. A. M. Roth, "Models of Authority, Hatshepsut's Predecessors in Power," in C. H. Roehrig, ed., *Hatshepsut from Queen to Pharaoh*, Figs. 1, 9.
25. W. S. Smith, *The Art and Architecture of Ancient Egypt*, revised by W. K. Simpson (New Haven: Yale University Press, 1981), Figs. 234–6 and p. 244 on affinity with Egyptians.
26. F. Dorman, "The Destruction of Hatshepsut's Memory: The Proscription of Hatshepsut," in C. H. Roehrig, ed., *Hatshepsut from Queen to Pharaoh*, 267, 269; D. Arnold, "The Destruction of the Statues of Hatshepsut," in *Hatshepsut from Queen to Pharaoh* (New York: Metropolitan Museum of Art, 2005), 270–76; and A. M. Roth, "Erasing a Reign," in C. H. Roehrig, ed., *Hatshepsut from Queen to Pharaoh*, 277–83.
27. C. Keller, "The Statuary of Hatshepsut," in C. H. Roehrig, ed., *Hatshepsut from Queen to Pharaoh*, 160.

Hatshepsut, Beloved of Amun—suffered greater destruction than her prenomen. This may be the result of attacks against the name Amun carried out during the Amarna period, but it may also be a reaction against the hieroglyph of a seated woman as pharaoh that formed part of her nomen. In addition, feminine grammatical markers were also hacked from her inscriptions.[28] That the feminine forms of the inscriptions, rather than feminine forms of statues, are systematically attacked could indicate that the discrepancy between image and reality was the disturbing factor. (Since the majority of Hatshepsut's images adopt a male form it is only the inscriptions that indicate her femininity.) No matter what sex the image presents, the inscription had to reflect her true identity so that the gods would recognize her. The pattern of erasure of those inscriptions suggests that it was indeed her biological gender that was upsetting. However, the question remains as to why such a long period (almost two decades) elapsed between the end of her reign and the destruction of her monuments by her successor Thutmose III.

Earlier scholarship focused on Thutmose III's supposed simmering resentment during his long co-regency. According to this theory, he finally erupted in angry retribution by ordering the destruction of her monuments and images. Recent discussions have stressed the fact that the defacements occurred at the *end* of his long reign rather than immediately after her death, pointing to a political rather than personal motivation for the destruction.[29] It has been suggested that erasing her memory helped to magnify his own achievements[30] or to stabilize his own succession.[31] The topic is still debated. The fact that Hatshepsut found it necessary to adopt male imagery remains, however, a key point, suggesting that her biological gender provided an important impetus for the destruction. Her successor, Thutmose III, returns to the use of traditional male/female color differentiation in his art.[32]

Despite Hatshepsut's early attempts to create a hybrid, male-female kingship, the ideology of kingship proves highly resistant to change. Pharaoh remains, at least symbolically, a male job. In fact, instead of changing the ideol-

---

28. A. M. Roth, "Erasing a Reign," in C. H. Roehrig, ed., *Hatshepsut from Queen to Pharaoh*, 277.
29. C. Keller, "Hatshepsut's Reputation in History," in C. H. Roehrig, ed., *Hatshepsut from Queen to Pharaoh*, 294–97, 281.
30. D. Arnold, "The Destruction of the Statues of Hatshepsut from Deir el-Bahri," in C. H. Roehrig, ed., *Hatshepsut from Queen to Pharaoh*, 274.
31. A. M. Roth, "Models of Authority: Hatshepsut's Predecessors in Power," 12, and "Erasing a Reign," 281, in C. H. Roehrig, ed., *Hatshepsut from Queen to Pharaoh*.
32. At least by the time of his successor Amenhotep II. See his Theban tomb (#92). Z. Hawass, *The Royal Tombs of Egypt* (London: Thames and Hudson, 2006), 51.

ogy, Hatshepsut ends up trying to confirm her place within the tradition by adopting all of the traditional male forms. The color convention is part of upholding this masculine tradition. During Hatshepsut's reign male/female color differentiation retains its symbolic function in supporting the traditional order in which the pharaoh's image, if not his inscriptions, is gendered male. The fact that skin color was one of the tools that she manipulated to legitimize her reign emphasizes the symbolic significance of color as gender indicator. Simple sun exposure is not the major factor determining the darkness or lightness of skin in Hatshepsut's images. The art of her reign confirms the close connection between male/female color differentiation and pharaonic ideology.

A similar link can be seen in the use of color in the art of the later New Kingdom Pharaoh Akhenaten, whose reign poses a slightly different question: What happens to male/female color differentiation when there is a major shift in ideology? Akhenaten changes the Egyptian pantheon and consequently the concept of the king's role within the cosmos. He shifts the capital of Egypt to a newly built city—Amarna, after which the distinctive art of the period is named. During the Amarna period new styles of depicting the human body are created. Among these is the abandonment of male/female color differentiation. While many of the monuments commissioned during Akhenaten's reign were destroyed during the restoration of the standard religion after his death, enough remains to show that men and women are painted the same color.[33] In some instances this color is closer to our orange, in others to the dark reddish brown previously reserved for men (as seen in Figure 10). Perhaps the most obvious example of this is the bust of Nefertiti, wife of Akhenaten, now in the Berlin Museum. While long admired as an icon of female beauty, this sculpture's orange skin color has received little attention, although this change marks a significant deviation from what had been the standard female color—yellow or white.[34] Two of the numerous examples of women's images using the new nontraditional palette include a head of a princess with a sidelock and a relief of Meritaten, another royal woman.[35]

33. There are a few instances of yellow stone used for female and at least one male image during this period. However, since even colored stones are often painted in Egyptian art this may not have been the final coloring of these pieces.

34. Aegyptisches Museum Berlin. J. Malek, *Egypt: 4000 Years of Art* (London: Phaidon Press, 2003), Figs. 190–91.

35. Princess with a side-lock, Louvre, Paris E 147.5, Relief of Kiya reworked for Meritaten, Ny Carlsberg Glyptothek AE IN 1776; R. E. Freed, Y. J. Markowitz, and S. H. D'Auria, eds., *Pharaohs of the Sun* (Boston: Bulfinch Press, 1999), Cat. No 57 and Cat. No. 46. Other examples can be found in C. Aldred, *Akhenaten and Nefertiti* (New York: Brooklyn Museum/Viking Press, 1973).

A number of freestanding sculptures of the royal women of Amarna are made from brown or red quartzite. It is tempting to add these to the list of examples of dark flesh for women, but the Egyptians were not averse to painting over colored stone. An early example is the Statue of King Menkaure and his wife from the Fourth Dynasty. The sculpture is made of a highly polished gray-black diorite, but clear traces remain of yellow paint for her flesh and red for his.[36] Thus, we cannot assume that the red color of the quartzite in the Amarna sculpture was necessarily the color of the finished piece.[37] One of the most often reproduced images from the Amarna period, a painting of two of the royal princesses in the Ashmolean Museum,[38] also has its own set of problems. In its current state the skin color of the two girls is a dark reddish brown, but the exact shade of this painting is problematic. Records show that the piece was varnished in the museum, darkening the colors. In addition, Petrie, the original excavator, remarks that orpiment, a yellow ochre, was removed during varnishing. Photos of the painting from its first exhibition show it to be considerably lighter.[39] The possibility remains that this could have been a yellow color or more likely a lighter orange equivalent to that of Nefertiti's bust in Berlin.

Dark paint for both male and female skin is also seen in works that were commissioned for non-royal individuals. A private stela found outside a house in Amarna shows two seated men (Menena and Yaya) facing two standing women (Tashety and Mery).[40] Aside from their names no further information is provided about their relationship or the occasion for the dedication. The men and the women are shown with the same brown-painted flesh.

Several factors need to be considered in attempting to determine why this change in a millennial-old iconographic formula occurs first and foremost in the new ideological framework presented by Akhenaten's replacement of the traditional gods of Egypt with worship of Aten, the solar disc, who was to be

36. Statue of Menkaure and Queen, Boston Museum of Fine Arts, Harvard University-Museum of Fine Arts Expedition, 11.17. 38. D. Arnold, K. Grzymski, and C. Ziegler, eds., *Egyptian Art in the Age of the Pyramids* (New York: Metropolitan Museum, 1999), Cat. No. 67, Fig. 50.

37. The same may hold for a yellow quartzite head of a princess from the Thutmose workshop at Amarna. Egyptian Museum Cairo. D. Arnold, L. Green, and J. Allen, eds., *The Royal Women of Amarna* (New York: Metropolitan Museum of Art, 1997), Fig. 51.

38. Princess Nefernefruaten-Tasherit and Nefernefurure. Arnold, Green, and Allen, eds., *Women of Amarna*, Fig. 49.

39. On the history and original color of this painting see F. Weatherhead, "Recording and Conservation of Painted Plaster from the Early Excavations at Amarna," in *Colour and Painting in Ancient Egypt*, ed. W. V. Davies (London: British Museum Press, 2001), 53–59.

40. Private stela from Amarna, San Diego Museum 14881. R. E. Freed, Y. J. Markowitz, and S. H. D'Auria, eds., *Pharaohs of the Sun*, 175.

worshipped to the exclusion of Egypt's previous multiplicity of deities. Akhenaten changes his own name; he was originally Amenhotep IV. Akhenaten, his new name, means beloved of the Aten. While there is much debate about the relationship between Akhenaten's religion and that of his father, Amenhotep III, the major alteration in Egyptian religion occurs under Akhenaten (Amenhotep IV). Amenhotep III did institute substantial changes to the Egyptian pantheon. He had himself deified and assimilated with the Aten, but the complete elevation of the Aten was Akhenaten's.[41]

While the Aten was the sole divinity of the Pantheon, pharaoh was the divine representative of the god on earth. As such, Akhenaten's image was uniquely linked with the sun disc. Depictions of the divinity clearly indicate that the particular manifestation worshipped is the divine light of the sun. The Aten is depicted as a disc from which rays ending in human hands extend. These hands and the disc are the same reddish brown color, traditionally used for males, that under Akhenaten was used for both males and females. The simplest explanation would then be that both male and female radiate with the light of the sun. The color also marks a direct symbolic link with the Aten himself. The disc, rays, and hands are all painted the same color as human flesh. The followers of Aten are thus visually linked with the deity through the use of color. Red, yellow, and gold were colors associated with the sun. Amenhotep III, Akhenaten's father and predecessor who began the emphasis on solar religion that was brought to full flower by Akhenaten, used stones in these colors for many of his statues.[42] Among these were the statues traditionally called the *Colossi of Memnon*. Made of golden quartzite, they flanked the entrance to his mortuary temple and were a focal point. Amenhotep III described these images as "rays . . . in people's faces like the sun-disc ('Aten') when it shines in the morning."[43] Here there would seem to be a clear association between color and the sun. Yet the color of these monuments is not the reddish brown and orange used for male and female in Amarna art. The quartzite is in fact closer to the

41. W. R. Johnson, "The Setting: History, Religion and Art," in Freed, Markowitz, and D'Auria, eds., *Pharaohs of the Sun*, 49. See also A. Kozloff, *Amenhotep III: Egypt's Radiant Pharaoh* (New York: Cambridge University Press, 2011), 250, who suggests that the new religion may have centered on the recently deceased Amenhotep III worshipped as the light of the sun.

42. A. P. Kozloff and B. M. Bryan, *Egypt's Dazzling Sun: Amenhotep III and His World* (Cleveland: Cleveland Museum of Art, 1992), 133. A. P. Kozloff, *Amenhotep III: Egypt's Radiant Pharoah*, 247.

43. M. Mallinson, "The Sacred Landscape," in Freed, Markowitz, and D'Auria, eds., *Pharaohs of the Sun*, Note 8, 74. The queens are also depicted in smaller form on these statues. A. P. Kozloff, *Amenhotep III: Egypt's Radiant Pharoah*, 126. He was also portrayed as Amun in a purplish red quartzite statue. P. Kozloff and B. M. Bryan, *Egypt's Dazzling Sun: Amenhotep III and His World*, 5.

traditional yellow for female skin. The rays of the sun as interpreted in art by Akhenaten are the reddish brown previously associated with male skin color, rather than the golden solar symbolism promoted by his father.

Akhenaten's "revolution" also had strong political effects, concentrating the power of the pharaoh while sharply curtailing that of the previously powerful priesthoods. As Kraus describes it, "Akehnaten's seventeen-year reign witnessed a revolution emanating from above that had as its political goal the concentration of absolute, unrestricted power in the crown."[44] This new ideology required artistic expression to materially embody its goals. Amarna style combines canonical modes of expression with new themes. The symbolic nature of Egyptian color use makes any change in male/female color differentiation an important part of any alteration in the message that elite monuments present. Reddish brown skin for both male and female is just one part of what is often termed an "artistic revolution" in which many of the previously established formulae of Egyptian art are altered. Amarna art is characterized by other changes, including a shift in the canon of proportions, an emphasis on informal "genre scenes" of the royal family, and an increase in the number of representations of the royal women as in the relief of two princesses in Figure 10.

An examination of these artistic alterations reveals a strong ideological framework behind the monuments. Among the most obvious artistic change is the representation of the pharaoh and members of his family. The physical characteristics and proportions displayed in his statuary are indeed different from what we might expect of a typical human being, let alone a pharaoh. All scholars have noted the unusual physical characteristics displayed in depictions of the Akhenaten, including spindly legs, elongated head, heavy chin, and flabby body. The most extreme examples are a series of colossal statues that lined the courtyard of a temple at Karnak called the *Gempaaten* ("Aten is found"). Six-meter-tall (twenty-foot) sandstone images of Akhenaten and possibly of his wife Nefertiti rest against the piers of the colonnade on the southern half of the west wall.[45] Somewhat smaller statues in red quartzite and smaller examples in black granite and red granite may have adorned the north side of this court. These statues have broad hips, full thighs and narrow shoulders, and

44. R. Kraus, "Akhetaten, a Portrait in Art of an Ancient Egyptian Capitol," in *Civilizations of the Ancient Near East*, ed. J. M. Sasson (New York: Hendrickson Publishers, 1995), 749.

45. H. Chevrier, "Rapport sur les travaux de karnak," 119–30; D. B. Redford, "East Karnak and the Sed-Festival of Akhenaten," in *Hommages à Jean Leclant I: Études pharaoniques* (Cairo, 1994), 485–87; Freed, Markowitz, and D'Auria, eds., *Pharaohs of the Sun*, Fig. 4 and Fig. 5.

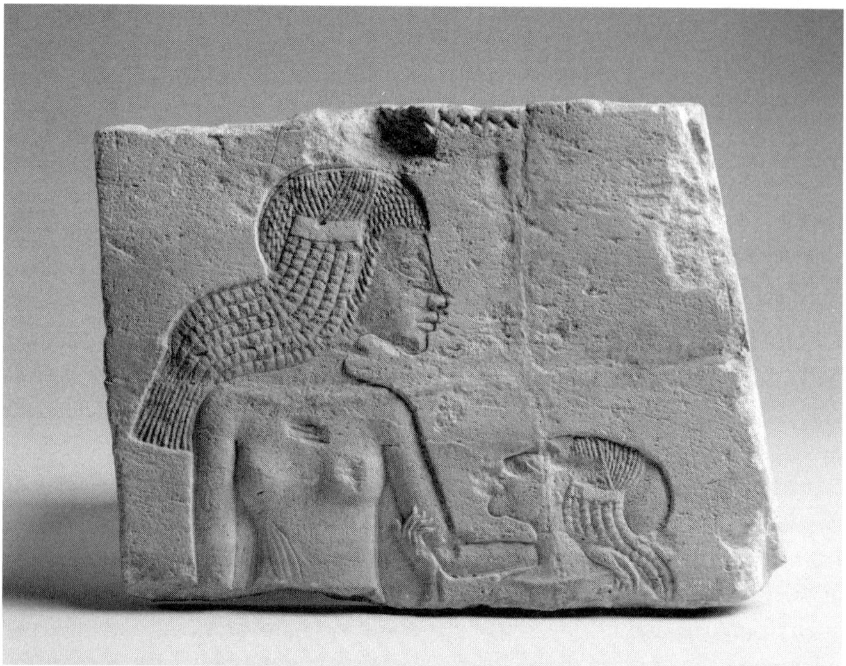

Fig. 10. Two princesses. Egypt, 18th dynasty, ca. 1353–1336 BC. Limestone, paint H. 8 3/4 in (21.2 cm); w. 11 ½ in (29.2 cm); th. 7/8 in (2.2 cm). (Gift of Norbert Schimmel, 1985 [1985.328.6]. Photo: Bruce White. The Metropolitan Museum of Art, New York, NY, U.S.A. Image copyright © The Metropolitan Museum of Art/Art Resource, NY.)

prominent buttocks. All of these features are usually female traits. This upper body voluptuousness contrasts with lower legs that are so spindly that they would seem unable to support the rest of the figure. The faces are elongated and have very prominent chins. In addition, Akhenaten is the first pharaoh to be portrayed consistently with pierced ears.[46] All of these features deviate from the strong, youthful, masculine physique traditionally found in representations of pharaoh. In particular, they seem to be skewed toward a more feminine body type.

The same exaggerated style is also found in relief sculpture showing the

46. A. Kozloff, "Sculpture: An Overview," in D. B. Redford, *The Oxford Encyclopedia of Ancient Egypt*, Vol. 3, 218–28.

royal family and in depictions of high government officials. Earlier scholars hailed these depictions as true likenesses representing the pharaoh's actual physique. According to this line of reasoning, everyone else was depicted in a similar style to emulate the pharaoh and perhaps mitigate any embarrassment over the king's strange appearance. In showing the king as he truly was, Amarna art was considered a kind of glorious burst of naturalism amidst the strict formality of previous Egyptian art. Stymied by a perceived grotesquery in his images, some have even sought explanations in glandular conditions. Scholars continue to debate whether these features have symbolic meaning or represent some kind of endocrine problem (Froelich's or Marfan's diseases, for example). Yet as a medium for the message of the ruling elite, Egyptian art does not necessarily conform to the true physical appearance of the pharaoh. Even when a pharaoh continues to rule at an advanced age, his images remain youthful. Another example of lack of conformity to the pharaoh's true physical type is found in the images of Hatshepsut. We have seen, for example, that indications of female anatomy were eventually eliminated from her images.

While Akhenaten's appearance seems radically different from his predecessors', Gay Robins has shown that it represents slight changes in the established grid system for designing the human figure. The preliminary step in carving a statue in Egypt involved marking all four sides of the block with a grid that set up a proportional relationship between the parts of the human body. During the reign of Akhenaten two grid squares were added at strategic locations to achieve the new proportions.[47] Length in face and neck were achieved by adding a square where the neck meets the shoulders. The drooping stomach was accommodated by adding a grid square to the torso. The traditional grid was thus expanded from eighteen to twenty. The legs appear short because of the added length of the rest of the body. In addition, statues of the pharaoh from early in his reign show him with standard rather than elongated proportions. A stele carved into the rock at Aswa shows the pharaoh instructing his chief sculptor Bak to create the new style.

Significantly, Akhenaten is shown with traditional proportions on one side and the elongated ones on the other. The presence of both clearly suggests that the change was not brought on by physical changes but because the pharaoh wished to promote a new ideology.[48] The stele documents the deliberate nature

47. G. Robins, *The Art of Ancient Egypt* (Cambridge: Cambridge University Press, 1997), 150–51.
48. R. Freed, "Art in the Service of Religion and the State," in Freed, Markowitz, and D'Auria, eds., *Pharaohs of the Sun*, 116, Note 22.

of the change in figure style. It shows both the change and the order for the change coming directly from the pharaoh.

That the new style of portraying the pharaoh fits his religious beliefs rather than physical deformities resulting from disease is also suggested by the fact that images created before his accession and the establishment of his new religious ideas conform to more standard pharaonic appearance[49] and traditional iconography. For example, while later in Akhenaten's reign Neferititi can be shown as equal in size to Akhenaten, in an earlier image in which he is still using his original name, Amenhotep IV, she was shown at a smaller scale than he. In addition, the exaggeration of physical features is modified in his later works.[50] This may reflect a relaxation of formulae after an early need to make a radical change to establish his ideas. Later, when his ideas had become standardized, he was able to modify these changes. The physical changes are thus a reworking of the old formulae for new ends.

The question remains as to how these artistic changes support and promote his message of Aten, the sun disc, as sole god. The Gempaaten colossi are a focus of this debate. Unlike Hatshepsut's representations, which always had either a clearly anatomically male or female body, many statues of Akhenaten seem to combine female physical characteristics with male. Despite the fact that several of the statues are nude, debate continues over whether they are meant to be images of Nefertiti or Akhenaten. The clothed figures wear the traditional male kilt and as with all representations of Egyptian males do not indicate the shape of the genitals beneath the fabric of the kilt. In all aspects of physiognomy the nude figures are identical to the clothed ones. This suggests a kind of divine bisexuality that would conform to the single all-encompassing nature of the Aten. In the Hymn to the Sun, the Aten is designated as both mother and father.[51] Therefore, images of the pharaoh would be a reflection of the bisexual nature of the god himself. If, however, the nude statues are Nefertiti, this identification becomes less tenable.

The fact that the regalia of the figures vary has been used to support yet another theory. Rita Freed among others suggests that they are images of the

49. Ibid., Fig. 74.

50. G. Robins, *Proportion and Style in Ancient Egyptian Art* (Austin: University of Texas Press, 1994). A. P. Kozloff, *Amenhotep III: Egypt's Radiant Pharaoh*, 45, suggests that the fact that his images become more traditional later in his reign indicates that the earlier forms were a deliberate choice.

51. "Hymn to the Aten," in M. Sandman, *Texts from the Time of Akhenaten* (Brussels: Fondation Egyptologique Reine, 1938), 93–94.

divine triad—Atum, Shu, and Tefnut—of the traditional creation story.[52] According to this theory, those wearing crowns represent the pharaoh in the guise of Atum, androgynous creator of the universe. Shu and Tefnut are represented by colossi wearing feather crowns and tall crowns, respectively. This identification is strengthened by an extraordinary detail that occurs in the rendering of the king's thighs and genital region. Traditionally, figures of kings and elite males wear opaque kilts that reveal nothing of what is underneath. By contrast, most two-dimensional figures of Akhenaten show the forward line of the near thigh beneath his kilt, as it runs upward to meet the stomach fold; no genitals are visible. This recalls the way in which fecundity figures are depicted. The pendulous stomach that the colossi also exhibit is a feature that can be connected with fecundity figures that are usually male and fat, in particular Hapy, the god of the Nile flood who is associated with Akhenaten in texts.[53] Like Akhenaten, they too show no genitalia, perhaps to enhance the notion of their corpulence through the conceit that the folds of the fat stomach droop so low as to conceal the genitals. This would argue against Akhenaten's figures as a combination of male and female since fecundity figures are usually gendered male.

If indeed these images are meant to invoke fecundity figures, they would fit one aspect of pharaoh's role—guarantor of the universe. Fecundity and fertility are significant aspects of promoting stability and order. While this similarity to fecundity figures is a possible explanation for the lack of visible male genitalia in the Gempaaten colossi, other statues indicate that this is not the entire story. The exaggerated features exhibited by the Karnak statues are modified in Akhenaten's later art toward more natural proportions so that the sharp contrast between the narrow upper body and the full stomach, thighs, and buttocks is mitigated, although these areas continue to be more prominent than in earlier art.[54] Perhaps Akhenaten chose this radical style as an announcement/precursor of his religious changes. By the time he moves the capital to his new city of Amarna, he may have fully established his principles and then introduces what is in fact an even more radical style, one in which the body is treated as much more of an organic whole.

---

52. R. Freed, "Art in the Service of Religion and the State," in Freed, Markowitz, and D'Auria, eds., *Pharaohs of the Sun*, 112.
53. G. Robins, *The Art of Ancient Egypt*, 150. For fecundity figures see J. J. Baines, *Fecundity Figures* (Chicago: Griffith Institute, 1985).
54. G. Robins, *Proportion and Style in Ancient Egyptian Art*, 15.

Yet, as we have seen, this art can be very formulaic, modifying but not totally abandoning traditional stylistic features. Where does color fit into these scenarios? If, in the early phase of his new religion, Akhenaten is in fact aiming for a bisexual depiction, male skin color would be a traditional element that he is retaining but modifying by combining it with rounded female physical features. In a similar fashion the grid pattern is altered but not abandoned to accommodate the new proportions. The question remains as to why women are now being depicted in the traditional male color scheme.

Clearly, with Hatshepsut the impetus for altering the color convention was the change from a male to a female occupant of the throne. During Akhenaten's reign Aten, the sun disc, replaces the original pantheon. Akhenaten changes traditional style in Egyptian art to convey this significant shift away from previous Egyptian religion. We need to ask how an alteration in the usual scheme of male/female color representation could be used to support and elucidate the new religion.

Akhenaten's religious revolution emphasizes worship of the Aten, the sun disc. All of the god's hands are painted the same dark color previously reserved for male flesh, a color that is now shared by everyone depicted in Amarna art. This might suggest that everyone is shown as browned by the rays of the sun. Or we could see it as a bold statement of the new religion's idea that the source of life is the rays of the sun disc, the Aten. So now we see everyone with skin darkened by those life-giving rays. We know that temples to the Aten had open courtyards flooded with sunlight rather than increasingly darker passageways leading to an inner sanctum, which was the usual style for temples.[55] Yet, as in discussions of the original color convention that limit it to a realistic depiction of indoors versus outdoors, this would again overlook the highly symbolic nature of Egyptian art that continues in the Amarna period.

As noted above, the change in the use of color is not the only break from tradition that occurs in Amarna art. The change in the color convention is but one part of a broader nexus that includes the other artistic changes that once again indicate a symbolic rather than a "realistic" interpretation. The Karnak temple reliefs include some scenes that had never appeared in temple contexts and that were subsequently employed at Amarna but seldom, if ever, again. These include vignettes of daily life, farm work, household activities, administration, and Nile scenes—all of which were previously standard only in private

55. P. Lacovara, "The City of Amarna," in Freed, Markowitz, and D'Auria, eds., *Pharaohs of the Sun*, 61–71.

tombs. This, combined with an unprecedented emphasis on the activities of the royal family depictions, gave Amarna art the appearance of naturalism. As Freed observes: "Whether recording royal expressions of emotion or showing streamers on a flagpole flying in the breeze, the art of Akhenaten focused on the here and now, capturing the moment like a snapshot."[56]

Amarna art is famous for "everyday" scenes of the king and queen in intimate poses with their daughters. Yet recent scholarship has suggested that rather than being casual "spontaneous" moments from the daily life of the palace, these scenes function as part of the iconographic message associated with the Aten. The royal family represents the fertility of the sun disc. There are no examples of anyone other than the royal family worshipping the Aten. Rather, everyone else "worshipped the royal family worshipping the disk."[57] The importance of the royal family as interpreters of the blessings of the Aten is illustrated in a change in funerary decoration. Tombs of high officials from the eastern cliffs at Amarna show that scenes of the royal family are substituted for the typical tomb scenes in which the deceased is shown supervising or participating in various everyday activities such as fishing and hunting.[58]

Akhenaten structured his new religion so that he and, to a lesser extent, his family—his wife Nefertiti and their daughters—were the intermediaries between the populace and the divine. Akhenaten, Nefertiti, and their daughters are shown in scenes that emphasize affection and intimacy. For example, a relief in Berlin shows a seated Akhenaten and Nefertiti facing each other beneath the rays of the Aten. Akhenaten is holding and kissing one of their daughters, while Nefertiti holds another daughter on her lap and another rests on her shoulder.[59] Such scenes of kissing and affection are unprecedented in Egyptian art.

There is also a profusion of depictions of the royal women, especially Nefertiti. A survey of the representations of elite women during this period shows that Nefertiti and her daughters enjoy an unprecedented status. In fact, some scholars have suggested that Nefertiti became co-regent. Scenes depicting Akhenaten alone are much less frequent than those in which Nefertiti and their daughters appear. Her name is written in two cartouches like that of a king. She is shown at least once wearing a crown almost identical to that of the pharaoh.

56. R. Freed, "Art in the Service of Religion and State," in Freed, Markowitz, and D'Auria, eds., *Pharaohs of the Sun*, 121.
57. Ibid.
58. Ibid.
59. Ägyptisches Museum Berlin. D. Arnold, *The Royal Women of Amarna*, Fig. 88.

In one of the ritual buildings at Karnak, tentatively identified as the "Mansion of the Benben Stone," only Nefertiti is present as the officiant in an offering scene.[60] Akhenaten is not present. At Akhetaten, his new capital city, some of the temples along the edges of the site may have been dedicated to the royal women.[61]

For the first time reliefs made major political statements about the queen's important role in affairs of state. The queen was depicted smiting enemies or in the presence of bound captives—iconography previously restricted to the king. At Amarna she is not shown as smaller than her husband.[62] The royal daughters, who numbered three by the time Amenhotep IV left Karnak, were also shown frequently.

The specific politics of power may be impossible to unravel given the fragmentary nature of the material recovered from Akhenaten's reign, but the fact remains that there is clear evidence of increased status for the queen at the same time as an equality of color is used. The fact that Akhenaten had no direct male heirs might suggest that the use of the previously male dark-brown color for the royal women is a subtle variation on the iconographical change attempted by Hatshepsut. Amarna women are painted brown and the pharaoh given "feminized features" to suggest that female rule is legitimate. Male skin color keeps the connotation of power associated with masculinity. Akhenaten could then designate one of his daughters or even Nefertiti as his successor.

This picture is complicated by what we know of the actual succession. Akhenaten seems to have named a male relative—Smenkaure—to rule after him. Smenkaure is a shadowy figure who seems to have died before he could assume the throne. Some scholars would like to see him as a masculinized version of Nefertiti.[63] If he were, in fact, Nefertiti in disguise, this reversion to a male successor would seem to go against the framework of feminine power set up during Akhenaten's reign, suggesting that he decided that the Egyptians would not accept a female ruler. As we have seen with Hatshepsut, while masculine representations of a female ruler might be accepted, actually saying that a woman was a man was not. It is, however, also possible that Smenkaure was the son of Akhenaten and Nefertiti.[64] If that is not true and the Nefertiti sce-

60. D. B. Redford, "The Beginning of the Heresy," in Freed, Markowitz, and D'Auria, eds., *Pharaohs of the Sun*, 58.
61. P. Lacovara, "The City of Amarna," in Freed, Markowitz, and D'Auria, eds., *Pharaohs of the Sun*, 64.
62. D. Arnold, "Aspects of the Royal Female Image," in D. Arnold, L. Green, and J. Allen, eds., *The Royal Women of Amarna: Aspects of Beauty from Ancient Egypt*, 85–93.
63. J. Tydesley, *Daughters of Isis* (London: Penguin, 1994), 236–37.
64. A. Kozloff, *Amenhotep III: Egypt's Radiant Pharaoh*, 250.

nario stands, it would be intriguing if, in the cases of Hatshepsut and Akhenaten, pharaoh had only female offspring. For Hatshepsut, "universalizing" the role of pharaoh would make it easier for her daughter to succeed her. Did Akhenaten learn from Hatshepsut and attempt to emphasize female power even more in his hybrid statues to pave the way for his daughters? Yet a closer look at the art of Akhenaten suggests that the promotion of the power of Nefertiti and of other royal women cannot be the sole explanation for abandoning male/female color differentiation during the Amarna period.

There have been other powerful women during times when the color convention was followed. During the reign of Amenhotep III, father of Akhenaten, Amenhotep's wife, Queen Tiy, is represented in inscriptions and art more than previous queens. Yet dark skin is not used for her representations before Akhenaten's ascension to the throne. A yellow jasper face in the Metropolitan Museum may represent Tiy in a pre-Amarna phase.[65] In an Amarna image she is shown with the dark male flesh color.[66] This suggests that the change is connected to something beyond an increasingly powerful role for royal women. The fact that, unlike Hatshepsut's use of male skin color in her images, male skin color during Akhenaten's reign is not confined to pharaoh or even to images of the royal family but is universal indicates that more is at work. We need to look at the religious ideology underlying Akhenaten's Amarna style for more clues to the lack of color differentiation during the Amarna period.

As others have noted, Nefertiti's role in the new religion was as a member of a new divine triad with Akhenaten and the Aten, mirroring the older and now discarded Creator god Atum and his male and female creations Shu and Tefenet. Now, Akhenaten and the royal family were the interpreters and transmitters of the blessings of the Aten. In the new religion the roles of male and female in guaranteeing the afterlife have changed from the old binary system with its consequent color coding to the Amarna doctrine expressing unity rather than duality. As Cheal suggests, the common color for male and female may also represent the "genderless time" before Atum created male and female.[67] The binary division serving as a clear and emphatic mark of difference was no longer necessary when a new religion placed the guarantee of fertility and the afterlife in the hands of the royal family, including not only the pharaoh but also

65. Fragment of a head of a queen, Metropolitan Museum N.Y.; D. Arnold, *Royal Women of Amarna*, Fig. 27.

66. See a wooden head from Medinet el-Gorub. Aegyptisches Museum und Papyrussammlung Berlin, 21834. Freed, Markowitz, and D'Auria, eds., *Pharaohs of the Sun*, Cat. No. 39.

67. C. Cheal, "The Meaning of Skin Color in Eighteenth Dynasty Egypt," in *Race and Identity in the Nile Valley*, C. Fluehr-Lobban and K. Rhodes, eds. (Trenton, NJ: Red Sea Press, 2004), 64.

the queen and royal daughters. The union of male and female was no longer the guarantor of the afterlife. The pharaoh and his family and their close relationship to the sun disc were. Male and female were united under the blessings of the Aten. Thus, females did not need to be marked any more as catalysts for creation by a separate color.[68]

Akhenaten's religious reforms did not survive his death. Without its supporting doctrine and with the return of the old theological system, the changed color scheme disappears, and the previously standard use of male/female color differentiation is re-instated.[69] Akhenaten's experiment emphasizes the ideological significance of color as gender indicator in Egyptian art. The use of contrasting dark/light colors and the brief use of a single color scheme are not simply conventions but evidence of great ideological significance for our understanding of ancient Egyptian society.

The reigns of Hatshepsut and Akhenaten clearly show that male/female color differentiation is closely connected to religious ideology. Hatshepsut uses the male color to bolster her legitimacy as pharaoh. During Akhenaten's reign a number of other changes occur in the artistic presentation of the pharaoh that suggest that a deeper symbolism, one involving changed ideological roles for male and female, may be involved. The switch to reddish brown for both males and females is but one of the many changes used to support the new ideology. As we have seen, color helps to promote Akhenaten's views about the correct ordering of the universe. Akhenaten abandons the female color to strengthen the claims of his religious changes. Both Hatshepsut and Akhenaten recognize and use the importance of color for getting across their particular messages. Clearly skin color is a major component of promoting and supporting distinctive pharaonic ideology. The importance of the deep traditional meaning of the color code as a message carrier is such that it can be modified for a time and purpose yet persist as an avatar of the Egyptian world view. Skin color in Egyptian art has far greater significance than sun exposure. It is part of the symbolic nexus that unifies Egyptian art.

---

68. On this point see M. A. Eaverly, "Colors of Power, Brown Men and Brown Women in the Art of Akhenaten," in *Colour in the Ancient Mediterranean World*, L. Cleland and K. Stears, eds. (Oxford: British Archaeological Reports, 2004), 53–55, 67.

69. See for example the painted reliefs from the Eighteenth Dynasty tomb of Horemheb. G. Robins, *The Art of Ancient Egypt*, Fig. 192.

CHAPTER 3

Greece

Establishing the Norm—the Road to Attic Black Figure

In the preceding chapters we have established that male/female color differentiation is an important signifier of gender roles in Egyptian art. Far from being a natural reflection of relative sun exposure it represents ideological difference. When it is not used in particular periods, such as during the reign of Akhenaten, or for particular individuals, such as Hatshepsut, that too is part of an ideological program. But can we say the same for Greece? How and why was this feature borrowed in the first place, and in what ways did it resonate with Greek and, in particular, with Athenian society, to become such a ubiquitous feature of Attic black figure? This chapter situates the Attic use of dark/light male/female color differentiation within the broader context of Greek and Athenian art in general, searching for underlying ideologies and social changes that may have brought about the adoption of this color differentiation. Unlike Egypt, Greece is not a single entity, nor is there a central authority overseeing artistic production and its message, so the search for answers will be even more complicated than in the preceding chapters, touching upon such big issues and hotly debated topics as the relationship of Dark Age society to Homer, the rise of the polis, and the origins of wall painting.

The earliest Athenian figural vase-painting style, Geometric, appears around 900 BC. Proto-Geometric, its predecessor, did not focus on figural decoration but instead relied on simple geometric shapes, such as circles and lines. Human figures were introduced only gradually but eventually became ubiquitous. These figures are themselves geometrized, reduced to dark silhouettes against a light background. Torsos are triangles, heads are circles, as we can see

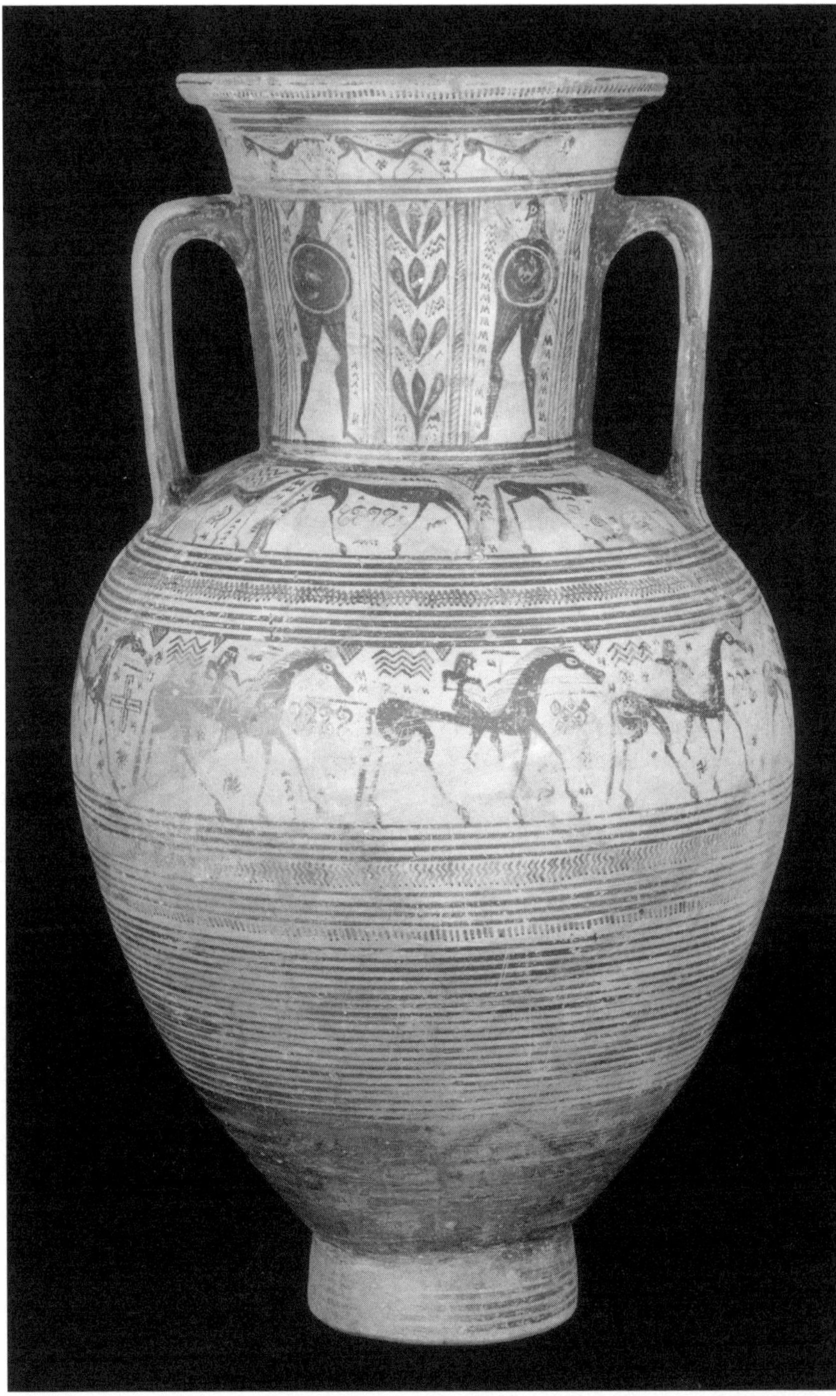

Fig. 11. Amphora. Greek, Early Orientalizing Period, 700–690 BC. Ceramic. Height: 41 1/8 in (104.4 cm); diameter 22 5/8 in (57.5 cm). (Museum of Fine Arts, Boston. Francis Bartlett donation of 1900, 03.782.)

in the lingering example of the style on a later vase in Figure 11. Significantly for our investigation, color is not used to distinguish between male and female.

This combination of stylized human figures and no male/female color differentiation would at first glance seem extraordinary in its departure from the figural style of the preceding Bronze Age Mycenaean frescoes, where in general women are painted white and men dark brown. These images themselves are heavily influenced by earlier Minoan frescoes, whose use of male/female color differentiation has usually been connected by Immerwahr and others to Egypt.[1] That the Minoans were in contact with the Egyptians is not doubted. There is ample evidence for political and trade connections between first Minoan Crete and, subsequently, Mycenaean Greece and Egypt. Inscriptions record actual visits, and figures in Minoan costume are shown carrying gifts in tomb paintings, especially during the New Kingdom.[2] Excavations at the site of Avaris have uncovered Minoan-style bull-jumping frescoes, painted by Minoan artists, on Egyptian soil.[3]

While many Bronze Age Greek frescoes follow Egyptian practice—men are painted dark brown and women white—there are exceptions that prove challenging to interpret. The "Toreador" fresco from Knossos, shown in Figure 12, provides the most striking case. The painting depicts bare-chested individuals wearing short kilts, a typically male costume, leaping over bulls. Yet two of the figures are painted white, the standard color for female skin. Because of this, the excavator, Sir Arthur Evans, identified these two—one standing behind the bull and the other preparing to grasp the bull's horns from the front—as women, and the third, a dark brown figure leaping over the back of the bull, as male.[4] However, the "women" display no female secondary sexual characteristics. Their kilts are more elaborately patterned than the "male" figure but are otherwise similarly short.

Much discussion surrounds the significance of the skin color in this scene.

---

1. S. A. Immerwahr, *Aegean Painting in the Bronze Age* (University Park: Pennsylvania State University Press, 1990); C. Gates, "The Adoption of Pictorial Imagery in Minoan Painting: A Comparativist Perspective," in A. P. Chapin, ed., *ΧΑΡΙΣ, Essays in Honor of Sara A. Immerwahr*, Hesperia Supplement 33 (Athens: American School of Classical Studies, 2004), 32.
2. E. H. Cline, *Sailing the Wine-Dark Sea: International Trade and the Late Bronze Age Aegean* (Oxford: British Archaeological Reports, 1994), discusses these interconnections and catalogs Egyptian objects in Crete. Cretans in an Egyptian tomb painting: Tomb of Senmut at Thebes. R. Higgins, *Minoan and Mycenaean Art* (London: Thames and Hudson, 1967), Fig. 187.
3. D. Preziosi and L. A. Hitchcock, *Aegean Art and Architecture* (Oxford: Oxford University Press, 1999), 193.
4. A. Evans, *The Palace of Minos*, Vol. I (London: Macmillan, 1921).

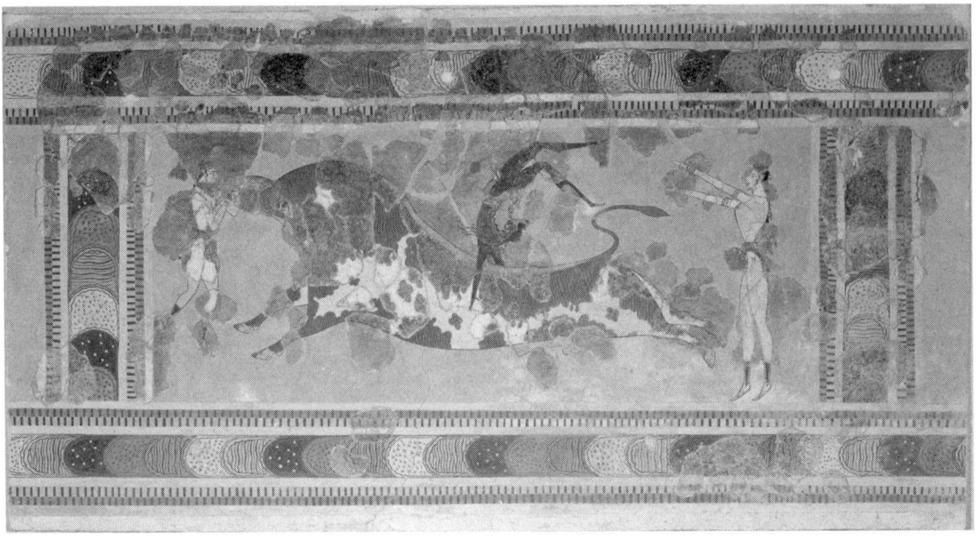

Fig. 12. Bull-leaping (Torreador fresco). From the palace at Knossos. Minoan, ca. 1450–1400 BC. (Archaeological Museum, Heraklion, Crete, Greece. Photo Credit: Scala/Art Resource, NY.)

There are four main theories: (1) that color serves as a temporal indicator to identify the progress of a single figure through the stages of bull jumping, much like stop-motion photography; (2) that some sort of rite of initiation for young males is shown in which their male identity would have emerged from the female; (3) that a ritual practice is depicted in which an ideologically significant identity switch between male and female would have occurred; or (4) that all figures are male with white being used to mark some figures as younger than others and thus undergoing some sort of initiation into the world of older males.[5] Without contemporary literary sources to aid in our interpretation, the exact meaning of the color of these figures remains elusive. However, the majority of frescoes in which color is gender specific militate against at least the time-lapse argument.

The picture is further complicated by Minoan and Mycenaean painting on

5. See D. Preziosi and L. A. Hitchcock, *Aegean Art and Architecture*, 169, for summary and relevant bibliography. On ambiguity see also M. C. Shaw, "The Priest King Fresco from Knossos: Man, Woman, Priest, King or Someone Else?" in A. P. Chapin, ed., *ΧΑΡΙΣ, Essays in Honor of Sara A. Immerwahr* (Princeton: American School of Classical Studies, 2004), 77–82, and N. Marinatos, "The Bull as Adversary: Some Observations on Bull-hunting, Bull-leaping," in *Ariadne: Festschrifft S. Alexiou* (Herakleion: Rethymnon, 1989), 23–32.

other media. With the exception of the elaborate stone Haghia Triadha sarcophus, neither Minoan nor Mycenaean sarcophagi (larnakes) follow the general fresco pattern of dark males and light females, although the shape and use of this type of burial equipment have been convincingly connected to Egypt.[6] The larnax figures are very schematic, but Mycenaean pictorial vases, an example of which is shown in Figure 13, provide more detailed figures with which to work. While not a huge corpus, these kraters, produced between 1400 and 1150 BC, share many themes with the frescoes—warfare, hunting, and so on—but do not use the dark/light skin color convention.[7] Instead, costume and secondary sexual characteristics (breasts for women, facial hair for men) indicate gender.[8] Although these women and men can be shown in long robes that cover the body, a greater variety of costumes (short tunic, leg guards, and boots) and equipment (spears and shields) indicates males. Female and male faces are painted in outline and left the reserved color of the clay.[9] There are, however, some examples that suggest that some form of color symbolism may be at work. When nude men are depicted, their bodies are completely filled in with dark paint although their heads are simply outlined.[10] The exposed limbs of clothed males are not treated in this way; they are drawn in outline and thus are the light reserved color of the clay.

Thus we have a stronger—although not always consistent—use of color to differentiate between men and women in the frescoes than in the vases. One might suspect that contrast between the two media is because of a limited color palette available to the vase painter. However, details of clothing are often painted in additional colors. The so-called Warrior Vase from Mycenae (13th c. BC), Figure 14, exemplifies such a use of extra colors.[11] On this vase a woman watches the departure of a row of warriors. Everyone is drawn in outline, and

6. Minoan Larnakes: L. V. Watrous, "The Origin and Iconography of the Late Minoan Painted Larnax," *Hesperia* 60, No. 3 (1991): 285–307; Mycenaean: E. Vermeule, "Painted Mycenaean Larnakes," *Journal of Hellenic Studies* 85 (1965): 123–48.

7. For these vases see E. Vermeule and V. Karageorghis, *Mycenaean Pictorial Vase Painting* (Cambridge: Harvard University Press, 1982).

8. On this point see L. Steel, "Women in Mycenaean Pictorial Vase Painting," in *Pictorial Pursuits: Figurative Painting on Mycenaean and Geometric Pottery, papers from two seminars at the Swedish Institute at Athens in 1999 and 2001*, ed. E. Rystedt and B. Wells (Stockholm: Svenska Institutet, 2006), 149.

9. See for example a krater in the Metropolitan Museum, Cesnola collection, purchased by subscription 1874–76 (74.51.966), in J. Mertens, *How to Read Greek Vases* (New York: Metropolitan Museum of Art, 2010), 40–43.

10. See for example a krater in the Metropolitan Museum, Cesnola collection, purchased by subscription 1874–76 (74.51.964). E. Vermeule and V. Karageorghis, *Mycenaean Pictorial Vase Painting*, contains many examples.

11. Athens National Museum 1426; E. Vermeule and V. Karageorghis, *Mycenaean Pictorial Vase Painting*, 130; D. Preziosi and L. A. Hitchcock, *Aegean Art and Architecture*, Fig. 123, 185.

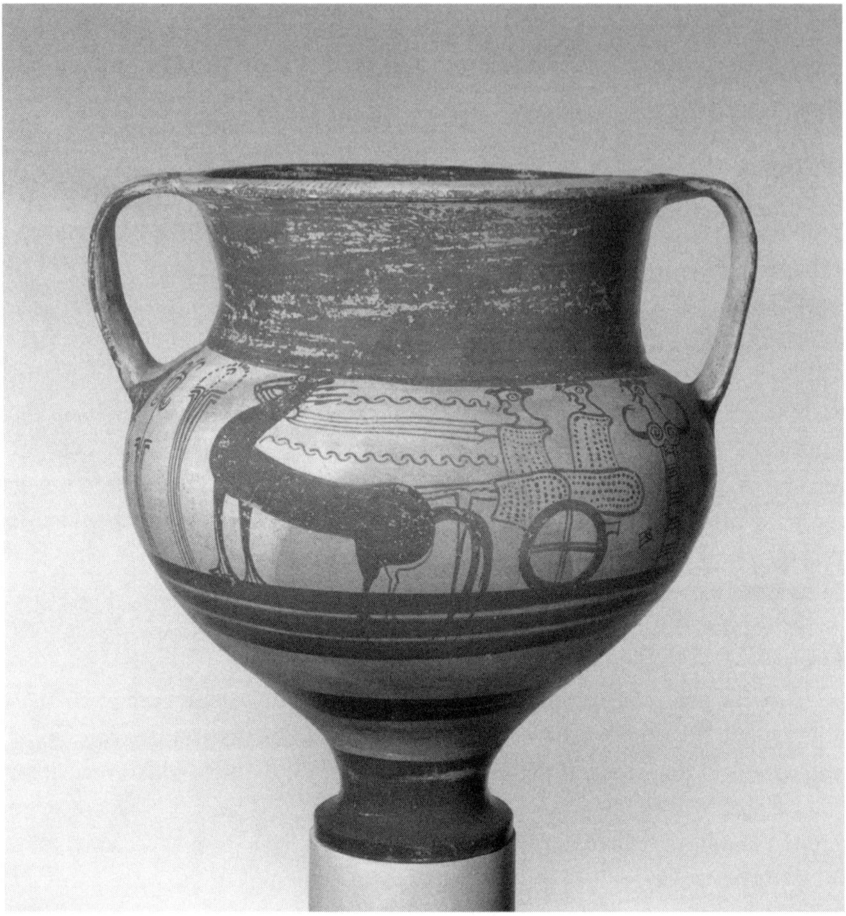

Fig. 13. Krater, ca. 1300–1230 BC. Terracotta, H. 13 3/8 in (41.6 cm), diameter 12 1/8 in (30.8 cm). Late Helladic IIIB Helladic, Mycenaean. (The Cesnola Collection, purchased by subscription, 1874–76 [74.51.966]. The Metropolitan Museum of Art, New York, NY, U.S.A. Image © The Metropolitan Museum of Art/Art Resource, NY.)

all flesh is reserved. The sole female on the vase stands out because of her costume, a long dress, in contrast to the warriors' short kilts and armor. In addition they are bearded. Her costume is decorated with a yellow-gold panel extending down the front. Other colors that have been noted on Mycenaean vases include dark brown and added white[12] but not for flesh color. Both of these models,

12. E. Vermeule and V. Karageorghis, *Mycenaean Pictorial Vase Painting*, 130.

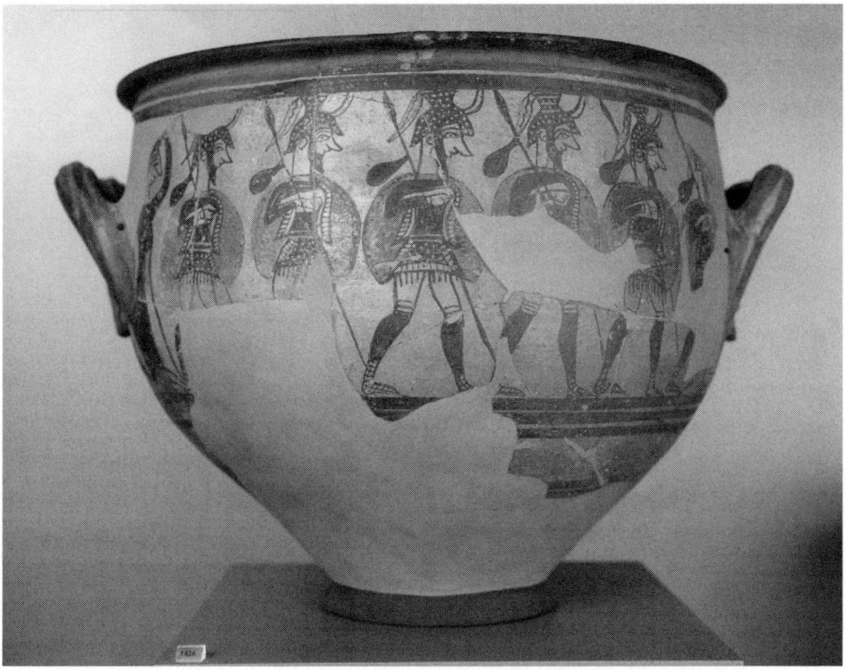

Fig. 14. Warrior vase. Mycenaean, 1300–1200 BC. From Mycenae. Terracotta, h. 16 in (41 cm) NM1426. (National Archaeological Museum, Athens, Greece. Photo Credit: Marie Mauzy/Art Resource, NY.)

frescoes and vases, may have been available to the Geometric artist for emulation, and they were not imitated. What they meant in their original context is another question and one that, based on the evidence that we have at hand, is not possible to answer. The two share the fact that men can be dark in frescoes as well as vases, although not always. Did the lack of color differentiation in vases result from a different gender ideology than that which pertained in the palaces? The exact relationship between the vases and the frescoes is debated. They share subject matter more than style.[13] Are Mycenaeans simply imitating Minoan frescoes because that is the style that "goes with" palaces, while the vases belong to a less palace-oriented tradition and express their own gender ideology rather than using Minoan forms? Are they expressing changes that

13. Ibid., 2, 5.

take place as the Bronze Age palatial world begins to decline? Again there is no clear answer.

While the Bronze Age ended in widespread destruction, the evidence from Dark Age objects found at Bronze Age tombs indicates that while the palace system had collapsed, all material traces of it were not obliterated.[14] Indeed, later Athenians prided themselves on having escaped invasion. Parts of the Cyclopean Mycenaean defensive wall on the Athenian Acropolis would still have been visible, although the palace that this wall protected is lost under the remains of the Classical buildings on the Acropolis.[15] Certainly parts of the Mycenaean past were still accessible to Dark Age inhabitants of Greece.

There is also evidence that contact with Egypt was not entirely lost during this period. While the collapse of the Mycenaean palace system did lead to disruption of trade, Egyptian and Near Eastern objects (scarabs, Isis figurines) found in geometric tombs indicate that all contact was not ended.[16] Geometric funerary vases, with their geometrized figural decoration, are found in graves that contained gold objects decorated with figures that show the full naturalistic forms used to depict humans in Egyptian and Near Eastern art.[17] Of course, because of the material from which they are made (blue faience or metal), many small-scale objects do not exhibit as wide-ranging a color palette as the monumental art found in those areas. However, some artistic features found in larger-scale non-portable art (art that would have had to have been viewed in situ) have also been detected. In particular, Benson noted a possible Egyptian prototype in one of the first figures depicted on many Attic Geometric vases, an image of a woman with upraised arms found above the handle on a vase in the Kerameikos.[18] Unlike her Late Geometric successors, she is nude and her body, while schematic, is much more rounded than is typical in Geometric art. Female nudity and rounded forms suggest Eastern influence, since female nudes are not the norm for Greek art until the fourth century BC. A nude

14. For the debate on the meaning of these deposits see C. M. Antonaccio, "Contesting the Past: Hero Cult, Tomb Cults and Epic in Early Greece," *American Journal of Archaeology*, 98, No. 3 (1994): 389–410. Whatever the purpose of the later objects found at these tombs, they do imply access.

15. J. Hurwit, *The Athenian Acropolis* (Cambridge: Cambridge University Press, 2000), 81–82, 88.

16. E. Guralnick, "The Egyptian Greek Connection in the 8th to 6th centuries BC: An Overview," in J. E. Coleman and C. A. Walt, eds., *Greeks and Barbarians: Essays on Interactions between Greeks and Non-Greeks in Antiquity and the Consequences for Eurocentrism* (Bethesda, MD: CDL Press, 1997), 127–54. Eastern objects were also found at Lefkandi (10th c. BC). See M. Popham, "An Engraved Near Eastern Bronze Bowl from Lefkandi," *Oxford Journal of Archaeology* 14 (1995): 103–7.

17. J. Hurwit, *The Art and Culture of Early Greece* (Ithaca: Cornell University Press, 1985), 67.

18. Kerameikos 1254. J. L. Benson, *Horse, Bird and Man* (Amherst: University of Massachusetts Press, 1970), 92.

Geometric ivory figurine from the Kerameikos, wearing a hat decorated with a meander, is usually assumed to be made of imported material and based on an eastern prototype.[19] The fact that the figure on the vase is a woman is made clear by the depiction of her breasts as two points projecting, in silhouette, from her left side.

This treatment, in admittedly much-less-schematic images of women, is also found in Egyptian tomb painting. Benson also suggests Egyptian influence as the source of the spatial arrangement of figures in funerary scenes on Geometric amphorae. He sees specific analogies between the hieratic poses in these scenes and the presence of a kneeling mourning figure often present beneath the bier.[20] Boardman, who remains skeptical, does point to possible Egyptian influence in the use (in Argive geometric) of wavy lines to indicate water and the placement of filling ornament in a manner similar to the use of determinative symbols in hieroglyphics, suggesting that these additional figures act to focus the meaning of a particular scene.[21] Thus, there is evidence to indicate that Egyptian art was available as a model and that certain aspects were borrowed. Significantly, however, male/female color differentiation was not adopted.

It is also not the case that gender ceased to be an important ordering principle in Athenian life during the Dark Ages. Gender-specific pottery shapes are used to hold the ashes of the deceased in Athenian Geometric graves. In male burials the handles on the ash-holding amphorae run vertically from the neck to the shoulder of the vase, and for women horizontally on the belly.[22] However, during this period a new post-palatial social order is emerging, and the fact that the artistic style is very different from either its predecessors, including Bronze Age artistic devices or contemporary Egyptian and Near Eastern models, indicates that none of these was deemed adequate to express the new norm. Indeed, Ian Morris suggests that the pattern revealed by Dark Age graves is one of deliberate rejection of Mycenaean models:

> Most of the choices being made by 1050 look like deliberate attempts to break with that past. Even if the basic skills needed to dig chamber tombs or build

19. Athens NM 776. J. Hurwit, *The Art and Culture of Early Greece*, Fig. 56, 128.
20. J. L. Benson, *Horse, Bird and Man*, 94–95.
21. J. Boardman, *Early Greek Vase Painting* (London: Thames and Hudson, 1998), 50.
22. J. N. Coldstream, "The Geometric Style: Birth of the Picture," in T. Rasmussen and N. Spivey, eds., *Looking at Greek Vases* (Cambridge: Cambridge University Press, 1991), 39.

> multi-room houses had somehow been forgotten, there were plenty of Mycenaean chamber tombs which could be re-used and houses which could at least be fixed up. Both things happened in the decades around 1100. But by 1050 most central Greeks distanced themselves from the past instead of trying to reproduce it.[23]

Thus Geometric stylized figures appear in a climate whose ideals cannot be expressed by the previous artistic style. Langdon has demonstrated a clear connection between Geometric art and the structure of Athenian society. She notes that in later Geometric vase painting women *and* men begin to be sharply differentiated. Costume and hairstyle became gender specific. Women are shown with long, flowing hair (which at least in Homeric verse is the sign of a maiden and not a mature woman, whose head is covered), and their long dresses are now belted.[24] This emphasis on costume as a way to differentiate male from female could represent a form of continuity with Bronze Age practice, since, as we have seen, some Mycenaean vases, such as the Warrior vase discussed above, did distinguish men and women in this way, while not distinguishing between them by color. However, while some themes, such as chariot images, do continue from the Mycenaean vase repertoire, the geometrized figure style is quite different from Bronze Age depictions.[25]

In addition, new scenes appear, in particular scenes of rows of men and women dancing and of men abducting women. Although landscape is never a major part of Geometric vase decoration, when vegetal elements are depicted they are most often associated with women, an indication perhaps of female liminality and of women as untamed occupants of the wild natural areas. Langdon correlates this new iconography and increasing differentiation with changes that can also be observed in burial practice. Namely, while earlier the wealthiest female graves were those of mature women, they are now those of younger women, and the associated grave goods are now connected with a premarital state. The loss of potential for the community in terms of fertility is acknowledged in these burials as well as the virginity of the deceased. They are supplied with equipment most suitable for a maiden, not a woman who has

23. I. Morris, *Archaeology as Cultural History: Words and Things in Iron Age Greece* (Malden, MA: Wiley-Blackwell, 2000), 206.
24. S. Langdon, *Art and Identity in Dark Age Greece* (Cambridge: Cambridge University Press, 2008).
25. On continuity of themes, see E. Rystedt and B. Wells, *Pictorial Pursuits: Figurative Painting on Mycenaean and Geometric Pottery*, 1.

borne children. The changed depiction correlates with societal change and works as part of, as Langdon puts it, "the construction of the maiden," the development of an ideology that places a premium on female virginity:

> Virginity burdened with family honor and gendered shame makes its entrance into Greek culture through these visual associations. . . . Her family's wealth and lineage, however limited, could be considerably enhanced by the girl's personal qualities—hence a new focus on purity, beauty, and exclusiveness, the elaboration of the *parthenos* as a social type.[26]

Understanding Geometric art as the visual manifestation of a cultural ideal helps explain the rejection of Bronze Age frescoes and the previously emulated Egyptian and Near Eastern representational prototypes for the human figure. The depiction of the human form in Geometric art is linked to the many societal changes that occur during the Dark Ages. Like Egyptian art it codifies gender relations.

Also like Egyptian art, the materials and the vocabulary of representation are in the hands of an elite group. In Dark Age Athens, of course, the ideology is not an integral part of a state-controlled religious and political bureaucracy. Instead, the images on Attic Geometric vases are part of a system of display that emphasizes the importance and wealth of families that have acquired power through the dissolution of the Mycenaean system of kingdoms. The locus of power has shifted from palace to household (*oikos*). With this new emphasis on clan and family a new iconography was developed, one that prized the implied reproductive and marriage alliance possibilities inherent in the *parthenos*.[27]

Male/female color differentiation is not part of this gender construction. As we have seen, other markers indicate difference between male and female. It is not a question of there not being a need to signify difference, but rather that the signifiers are not as dramatic as contrasting skin color. Superficial elements such as clothing and hairstyle indicate social status and age, but not the fundamental difference that color implies. (Theoretically a man could wear a dress or grow his hair long.) While more attention has been paid to the fact that this period's multi-figure scenes lay the groundwork for the later exploitation of narrative that is to become a hallmark of Athenian vase painting, it is worth

26. S. Langdon, *Art and Identity in Dark Age Greece*, 196.
27. Ibid., 130.

noting that the idea of depicting ideal gender relations is also an important part of the renewal of figural style that marks the Geometric period.

Later, when male/female color differentiation is re-adopted in Greece it is in response to another set of societal changes. This re-adoption takes place against the broad backdrop of the embrace by aristocratic elites of the East as the standard for luxury that occurs in the eighth and seventh centuries BC, traditionally called by scholars the *Orientalizing period.*[28] In vase painting this manifests itself in the use of composite animals and floral patterns whose original home is the Near East. Throughout Greece some city-states seem receptive to incorporating Eastern-inspired motifs, and some do not.[29] Corinth, among the most receptive cities, creates Proto-Corinthian, a miniature vase-painting style with heavy reliance on Near Eastern animals. Eventually the Corinthians develop a more rounded human figure type that replaces Athenian Geometric as the dominant figure style. Athens eventually produces Proto-Attic, a decorative style emphasizing large figures and narrative scenes.[30]

Trade, particularly by Phoenician merchants, has long been considered a major conduit for the transmittal of these styles between Greece and the East.[31] However, re-examinations of the question of Phoenician traders have shown that they were not necessarily the only conduits for material from Assyria and Egypt. Gunter has recently shown that the trade model simplifies what was a complex relationship of visitors, traveling artisans, displaced populations, and other forms of contact that occurred under the umbrella of the Neo-Assyrian Empire. Gifts from the Assyrian center to provincial governors and to ruling elites in other parts of the empire played a part in the accessibility of Assyrian art.[32] Motifs could have been spread through imported objects but also through firsthand impact when traveling Greeks saw Near Eastern monuments.

While the Near Eastern–influenced Corinthian vases are widespread, Athenian Proto-Attic vase painting is much more limited in number and distribution. Whitley has identified Athenian use of Orientalizing motifs as a "ration-

28. This term has been recently called into question because of its polarizing emphasis on an East-West dichotomy. See for example G. Hoffman, *Imports and Immigrants: Near Eastern Contacts with Iron Age Crete* (Ann Arbor: University of Michigan Press, 1997), 2, and A. C. Gunter, *Greek Art and the Orient* (Cambridge: Cambridge University Press, 2009), 5. I use it understanding its drawbacks but accepting its convenience in light of its years of traditional use in scholarship.

29. On this point see J. Boardman, *Early Greek Vase Painting*, 84.

30. For Proto-Attic pottery see G. Rocco, *La ceramografia protoattica: pittori e botteghe (710–630 a.c.)* (Rahden/Westff: VML, Verlag Marie Leidorf, 2008).

31. The major work on the topic is S. P. Morris, *Daidalos and the Origins of Greek Art* (Princeton: Princeton University Press, 1992).

32. A. C. Gunter, *Greek Art and the Orient*, 5.

ing" brought about by the elite who maintain their status by appropriating the eastern style for their own monuments.[33] These vases are not in the majority in any of the places where they are found, but in Athens they are almost entirely restricted to burials in the Kerameikos, the same location where earlier the large Geometric vases were used as grave markers for elite burials.

Neither Proto-Corinthian nor Proto-Attic initially uses dark/light male/female color differentiation. In early Proto-Corinthian vases, figures are drawn in outline, and thus both men and women are the light color of the fired clay. Some Proto-Attic vases, the Black and White group, used added white paint for men and women.[34] There are occasional examples of men painted in dark silhouette on proto-Attic vases with faces left in reserve that suggest a possible iconographic significance for the dark color. For example, on one side of a single vase, a krater from Aegina by the Oresteia Painter, we can have male figures with white skin and other male figures painted as dark silhouettes and on the other side a female figure shooting arrows (Artemis?) with an outline face and dark silhouette arms.[35] S. P. Morris suggests that white in the work of the Oresteia Painter "makes a symbolic distinction between conqueror and captive."[36]

However, this distinction does not apply to all Proto-Attic vases as we can see by examining a vase by the Polyphemos Painter Amphora from Eleusis, shown in Figure 15.[37] Here, unlike the Oresteia Painter vase, we can clearly identify the scenes and figures depicted. There are two recognizable scenes on this vase, the blinding of Polyphemos, and Perseus fleeing from the Gorgon. Thus we might expect to be able to connect color to iconography. Looking first at the Cyclops episode, on the neck of the vase, we see Odysseus and three companions blinding Polyphemos with a stake. Odysseus' companions are painted in dark silhouette except for their faces, which are drawn in outline. The hero's body is outlined in black. The outline is not one continuous line but a series of contouring brushstrokes. His flesh is painted white. The Cyclops is painted in the same black silhouette with outline face as Odysseus' companions.

One is reminded of the silhouette bodies and outline faces of nude male

33. J. Whitley, "Proto-Attic Pottery: A Contextual Approach," in *Classical Greece: Ancient Histories and Modern Archaeologies*, ed. I. Morris (Cambridge: Cambridge University Press, 1994), 58.

34. The major study of these vases is S. P. Morris, *The Black and White Style: Athens and Aegina in the Orientalizing Period* (New Haven: Yale University Press, 1994).

35. Attic krater from Aegina: Berlin A 32, by the Oresteia Painter. S. P. Morris, *The Black and White Style: Athens and Aegina in the Orientalizing Period*, No. 2, Pl. 13; J. Boardman, *Early Greek Vase Painting*, Fig. 209.

36. S. P. Morris, *The Black and White Style: Athens and Aegina in the Orientalizing Period*, 59.

37. Eleusis Museum. S. P. Morris, *The Black and White Style: Athens and Aegina in the Orientalizing Period*, No. 8, 122; J. Boardman, *Early Greek Vase Painting*, Fig. 209 and cover.

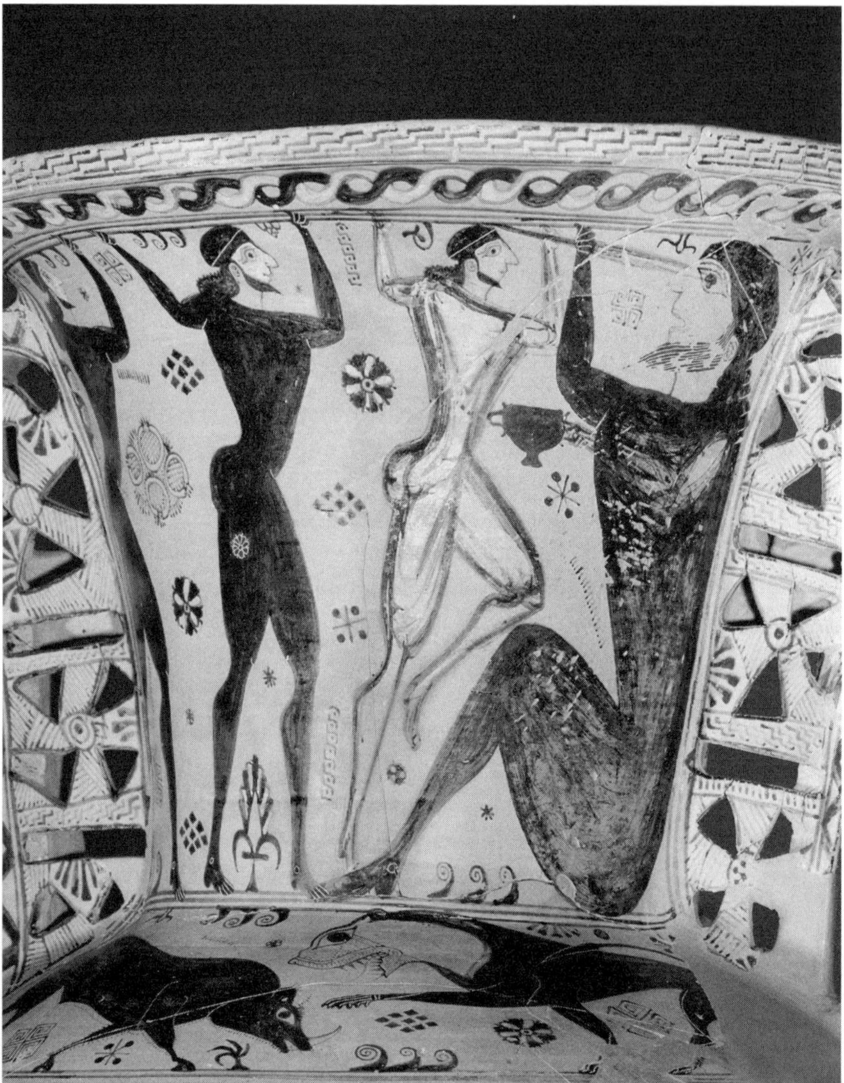

Fig. 15. Early Attic amphora. Seventh century BC. The blinding of Polyphemos. (Archaeological Museum, Eleusis, Greece. Photo Credit: Erich Lessing/Art Resource, NY.)

figures on Mycenaean pictorial vases that sometimes exhibited a similar treatment. The Orientalizing period is marked by an increase in artifacts left at Bronze Age tombs.[38] The connection between the rise of mythological themes and the development of Homeric epic is debated, but most scholars agree that during the Orientalizing period Greeks are engaged in formulating or celebrating a mythic past.[39] Emulation of an earlier figural style could be part of that process.

What, however, are we to make of the added white color for Odysseus? This is not part of either the Bronze Age fresco or pictorial vase-painting tradition. Explanations have tended to narrowly focus on what meaning might apply to this particular episode, rather than looking within the broader context of color in Proto-Attic vase painting. So, for example, Odysseus' color has been explained as a sign that the Cyclops cannot see him or that he is light because he is the protagonist.[40] Objections can be raised to both of these explanations. If invisibility is the key factor, why are the companions, who are helping Odysseus, not also painted the "color of invisibility"? Arguing against the age explanation is the fact that at least in later vase painting a beard is the sign of maturity, and Odysseus and his companions all have beards. Another suggestion is that he is white because he is the hero. Yet on the belly of the same vase, Perseus, the hero of the Gorgon-slaying episode, is painted with black skin like Odysseus' companions. The Gorgons, who are female, are painted white. Is there a clear pattern to the use of color for flesh in this vase? The only clearly discernible (at least to us) pattern among all the vases is that men are shown as both dark and light, with the light often being provided by an additional layer of white paint, while women are almost never shown as dark.

The use of white for male skin color in these vases conforms not to the Egyptian model but to the art of Assyria. While we do not have a large volume of painting preserved from Assyria, what we do have shows men painted white. In fact, a well-preserved example, the eighth-century-BC wall paintings from the provincial governor's house at Til Barsip (Tell Ahmar), shows white for

38. I. Morris, *Archaeology as Cultural History: Words and Things in Iron Age Greece*, 267.

39. There is a huge bibliography on this topic. See, for example, J. M. Hurwit, *The Art and Culture of Early Greece*, 21, and I. Morris, *Archaeology as Cultural History: Words and Things in Iron Age Greece*, 267.

40. For emphasis on protagonist, see G. Ferrari, "Menelās," *Journal of Hellenic Studies* (1987): 107; (1985): 181; Hurwit, *The Art and Culture of Early Greece*, 169; I. Scheibler, "Features and Intentions of Color-Schemes in Archaic Vase-Painting," in *Color in Ancient Greece: The Role of Color in Ancient Greek Art and Architecture (700–31 BC)*, ed. M. A. Tiverios and D. S. Tsiafakis (Thessaloniki, 2002), 65; Invisible: R. Osborne, *Archaic and Classical Greek Art* (Oxford: Oxford University Press, 1998), 60. Emphasis: C. Smith, "A Proto-Attic Vase," *Journal of Hellenic Studies* 22 (1902): 36.

male and female skin.[41] In some of these paintings the king is shown in various depictions receiving an audience. He and all of his attendant courtiers are shown with white skin. No women are present in these scenes. However, two women are present in another painting from the same palace in which Assyrian soldiers are shown executing prisoners, and these women too are painted white.

The exact color scheme of the sculpted reliefs from the palaces of the Assyrian kings is difficult to determine. Early excavators also describe white paint on the male figures from the relief sculptures of these palaces. When paint is preserved it is usually found on the eyes and hair, and enough paint was preserved on reliefs excavated at Nimrud in the 1950s to show that beards, hair, rims of eyes, and pupils were painted black. The whites of the eyes were painted white, and jewelry was picked out in yellow, presumably to indicate gold. Glazed bricks from Nimrud showing the king standing between two attendants and holding a bow have traces of red paint on sandals of some figures and on the king's bow.[42] Looking farther back in time we can see that the Near East has a history in which there does not seem to be a strict adherence to differentiating male and female by color. Although very little wall painting from this area survives, what is preserved does not show a skin color contrast between men and women. Monumental wall paintings from several large rooms and courts at the Palace of King Zimri-Lim at Mari (ca. 1760 BC) include scenes of warfare and worship as well as some that may show aspects of daily life.[43] In only one instance is exposed flesh, male or female, not painted brown. In the lowest- and smallest-scale register, a man carrying fish has white skin. A fragmentary figure to the left in the same pose, but with brown skin, suggests that this lowest register might show an alternation of light and dark male figures forming a decorative pattern that echoes the border above these figures—a pattern of alternating red and white diamonds. In this case the color would be purely decorative, something that is also observed in Egypt where, as we have seen, figures that overlap in a group scene are often painted in alternating light and dark shades of the standard reddish-brown male color. However, in the main panels of the Mari painting in which the king is shown in the company of goddesses (identifiable from their hairstyle, costume, and headdress) offering libations to a seated male god and in another panel in which the goddess Ishtar receives an offering made by another goddess, no color distinction is made between male

41. A. Parrot, *Ninevah and Babylon* (London: Thames and Hudson, 1961), Figs. 344–47.
42. D. Collon, *Ancient Near Eastern Art* (Berkeley: University of California Press, 1995), 136.
43. A. Parrot, *Ninevah and Babylon*, Figs. 344–47.

and female flesh. All skin is painted brown. The same holds true for another of the Mari paintings, the so-called Investiture scene. A male figure, presumably Zimri-Lim, is shown touching emblems of rule handed to him by the goddess Ishtar. In the register below, two goddesses holding flowing vases are also painted brown. As Spycket notes in her discussion of the statuette of Ur Nansh of Mari freestanding sculpture, it is often difficult to differentiate between male and female. Neither hairstyle nor costume is always definitive.[44] In the case of that statue, comparisons with the hairstyle and costume of male statues favor the identification of the statue as a man. The skin is painted dark, but the statue's only inscription is the name of a woman from Mari.

This far-from-exhaustive survey of Near Eastern art suggests that while the flesh of figures could be painted, color was not used as a gender signifier. We have seen examples in which male and female figures in the same painting are reddish brown (Mari) and examples in which both are white (Til Barsip). Are there underlying reasons for not contrasting men and women through color in the Near East? Unlike Egypt, Mesopotamia was not a single political entity but a series of successive and sometimes overlapping civilizations. Still, some general principles seem to hold throughout the region, although the evidence is admittedly fragmentary. Intriguingly, some features suggest a different concept of gender than that operating in Egypt. If we look at the early Sumerian civilization (3500–2340 BC), language reveals this. Rather than distinguishing grammatically between male and female, Sumerian has a single gender—"human"—and the word for deity is similarly not marked for gender. The names of gods as well as goddesses are formed from the word *nin* and a place-name. Asher-Greve notes that Mesopotamia does not follow the "Graeco-European tradition" that inscribes the mind/body dichotomy with two binary gender categories assumed to be universal: male mind versus female body."[45] S. Pollock and R. Bembeck's study of Sumerian cylinder seals shows that gender may not have been a binary concept for the Sumerians. Human images on the seals can be divided into four categories: men, women (both clearly marked by primary or secondary sex characteristics—penises, beards, breasts), pig-tailed figures

---

44. A. Spycket, *La Statuaire du Proche-Orient ancien* (Cologne: Brill Academic Publishers, 1981), 93–95; Z. Bahrani, *Women of Babylon: Gender and Representation in Mesopotamia* (London: Routledge, 2001), 103.

45. J. G. Westenholz, "Goddesses of the Ancient Near East 3000–1000 BC," in *Ancient Goddesses*, ed. L. Goodison and C. Morris (Madison: University of Wisconsin Press, 1998), 68. J. M. Asher-Greve, "The Essential Body: Mesopotamian Conceptions of the Gendered Body," in M. Wyke, ed., *Gender and the Body in the Ancient Mediterranean* (Oxford: Blackwell Publishers, 1998), 8.

(hairstyle and costume usually associated with women), and naked hairless individuals with no identifying characteristics, which the authors suggest may represent a third gender category.[46] Thus anything that marks a sharp binary division between male and female would not be appropriate. Male/female color differentiation does not fit with a world view that does not emphasize dichotomy. While, unlike the seals, the dearth of female images, other than goddesses, in the monumental art of Mesopotamia[47] might suggest that there was no need to sharply mark contrast, the fact that such a contrast would not express underlying ideas about gender is more telling. Assyria thus provided an influential artistic source for Orientalizing Greek vase painting, but in the middle of the seventh century Egyptian-style male/female color differentiation reappears in Greece in a style of vase painting generally referred to by scholars as *polychrome*. The production and distribution of these vases are limited. Examples are present in the vase painting of Argos, Naxos, Melos, Megara Hyblaea, Crete, the Cyclades, and Attica.[48] With the exception of Melos, where polychrome vases appear a few decades later, all of these wares appear rather suddenly in mid-seventh century BC and do not continue much beyond that period. These polychrome vases provide the first examples of male/female color differentiation in the Egyptian style—dark reddish brown men and white women—in Greek art since the Bronze Age. The term *polychrome* is somewhat misleading since the palette is not broad, primarily red, white, yellow, and some blue. Important, however, is the use of a brown paint wash for male flesh, not a black-painted silhouette or outline with the flesh reserved as had previously been used. This striking feature is most prominent on Proto-Corinthian vases, where more complex figure scenes are also introduced along with the development of a new style of vase painting, namely, black figure, in which black for outline and sil-

46. S. Pollock and R. Bembeck, "And They Said, Let Us Make Gods in Our Image: Gendered Ideologies in Ancient Mesopotamia," in *Reading the Body*, ed. A. Rautman (Philadelphia: University of Pennsylvania Press, 2000), 155.

47. On the absence of non-divine women, see I. Winter, "Women in Public: The Disk of Enheduanna, the Beginning of the Office of EN-Priestess and the Weight of Visual Evidence," in *La Femme dans le Proche-Orient Antique*, ed. J. M. Durand (Paris: Rencontre Assyriologique Internationale, 1987), 189–201, and S. Pollock, *Ancient Mesopotamia: The Eden that Never Was* (Cambridge: Cambridge University Press, 1999), 181.

48. G. P. Schaus, "The Beginning of Greek Polychrome Painting," *Journal of Hellenic Studies*, 108 (1988); N. J. Koch, *Picturae Initiis: Die Anfange der Griechischen Malerei im 7. Jahrhundert v.Chr.* (Munich: Biering & Brinkmann, 1996); J. A. Papapostolou, "Colour in Ancient Painting," in Tiverios and Tsiafakis, eds., *Color in Ancient Greece: The Role of Color in Ancient Greek Art and Architecture 700–31 BC*, 53–64; I. Scheibler, "Features and Intentions of Color-Schemes in Archaic Vase-Painting," in M. A. Tiverios and D. S. Tsiafakis, eds., *Color in Ancient Greece: The Role of Color in Ancient Greek Art and Architecture*, 65–75.

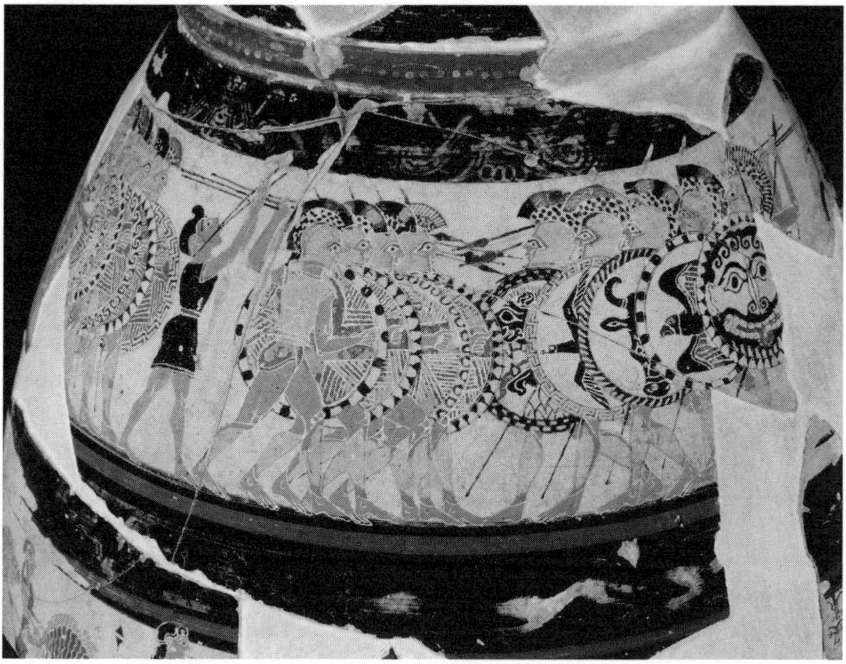

Fig. 16. Chigi vase. Detail of Hoplites. Oenochoe (wine pitcher) from Corinth. Proto-Corinthian style, middle seventh century BC. Height 10 1/14 in. (Museo Nazionale di Villa Giulia, Rome, Italy. Photo Credit: Scala/Art Resource, NY.)

houette is no longer created through added paint but through the firing process, leading to a shinier and more durable image.

The most famous example is the Chigi Olpe, shown in Figure 16.[49] While the torsos of the male figures on these vases are the shiny black typical of black figure, their faces and exposed limbs are drawn in outline (using the same clay slip used for the torsos). Their flesh is, however, painted in a brown wash. These are not the white males of Assyria but rather the reddish brown men of Egypt. Women are drawn in outline. While, as we shall see, there are few depictions of women on Corinthian vases, female flesh is indicated by a layer of added white paint over the fired white of the regular clay surface as on three goddesses in the

49. Rome Villa Giulia 22679. J. Boardman, *Early Greek Vase Painting*, 94–95 and Fig. 178, 1–3; J. Hurwit, "Reading the Chigi Vase," *Hesperia* 71, No. 1 (2002): 1–22.

Judgment of Paris scene depicted on the olpe. The brown wash for male flesh is also found on a series of terracotta plaques, with mythological themes that served as architectural decoration on the Temples of Apollo at Thermon and Calydon.[50] Debate rages over whether these architectural plaques and the polychrome vases are copying or at least influenced by the contemporary wall painting of which we have no trace other than mentions in ancient authors. Our exploration of male/female color differentiation cannot answer that question. For our purposes it is sufficient to say that the vases indicate the probable skin-color palette for such paintings.

This is also the period when large-scale stone sculpture becomes a part of the Greek artistic repertoire after a hiatus during the Dark Ages. The role of Egypt in the development of early Greek sculpture is generally accepted, although a recent re-evaluation has shown that early male figures, kouroi, do not conform as strictly to the Egyptian canon of proportions as was once thought.[51] However, other factors, such as the colossal size of the early statues and the use of Egyptian-style stonecutting tools, strongly support Egypt's role. In addition, kouroi adopt a stance very similar to Egyptian figures. The use of skin color differentiation in sculpture would also be a further connection between early Greek sculpture and Egyptian influence. However, few of the Greek pieces retain their original paint. Recent technological advances promoted by the work of V. Brinkmann have allowed even more paint to be recovered, and it is clear that the sculptor's color palette included red, yellow, green, blue, purple, and orange. Indeed, some sixth-century BC male sculpted images do have traces of reddish-brown paint,[52] although nothing as early as the polychrome vases shows this use in color.

The pharaoh Psammetichus I (664–610 BC) recruited East Greek and Car-

50. J. A. Papapostolou, "Colour in Ancient Painting," in M. A. Tiverios and D. S. Tsiafakis, eds., *Color in Ancient Greece: The Role of Color in Ancient Greek Art and Architecture*, 53–64; 61; K. Shefold, *Myth and Legend in Early Greek Art* (New York: Harry N. Abrams, 1966), 35 and Pls. 18–21.

51. On connection to Egypt, see B. S. Ridgway, *The Archaic Style in Greek Sculpture* (Chicago: Ares Publications, 1993), 21; for the re-evaluation of the relationship of the Egyptian canon to Greek sculpture, see J. A. Carter and L. J. Steinburg, "Kouroi and Statistics," *American Journal of Archaeology*, 114, No. 1 (2010): 103–28.

52. For example, the poros pediments from the Acropolis. V. Brinkmann, "Die Farben der Archaischen und Frühklassischen Skulptur," in *Bunte Götter, Die Farbigkeit Antike Skulptur*, ed. V. Brinkmann (Munich: Biering & Brinkmann, 2004), 35, No. 6, 7, and 8; V. Manzelli, "La Policromia Nella Statuaria Greca Arcaica," *Studia Archeologica* 69 (1994): 183–84; V. Brinkmann, "Die Polychromie der Archaischen und Frühklassischen Skulptur," in *Studien zur Antiken Malerei und Farbgebung* 5, ed. R. Biering and V. Brinkmann (Munich: Biering & Brinkmann, 2003), 43. No. 6 Bluebeard pediment, Nos. 7 and 8 Introduction pediment; Siphnian Treasury: No. 95, 122; B. S. Ridgway, *Prayers in Stone, Greek Architectural Sculpture* (Berkeley: University of California Press, 1999), 110, poros pediments.

ian mercenaries, thus paving the way for further trade and the right of Greeks to settle in Egypt,[53] and this kind of contact allowed firsthand exposure to the colors of Egyptian painting on freestanding sculpture and on building walls, which could not have failed to make a strong impression on Greek viewers, just as the colossal scale of these monuments influenced the development of monumental sculpture in Greece. Contact, however, cannot be the sole explanation for the use of male/female color differentiation in both the architectural plaques and the polychrome vases. As we have seen, there was contact with the Near East and Egypt during the Geometric period, yet the convention was not used as part of Greek decorative schemes. It was not an effective device for expressing Greek gender ideology. Male/female color differentiation must resonate with themes in Greek society in order to be something worth incorporating.

This is also, as it is often called, the *Age of Homer*, the period in which writing re-emerges and is first used to record poetry. Homer and Hesiod indicate underlying themes that male/female color differentiation would be the ideal vehicle to express. Homer describes men as dark and women as white. That this reflects a symbolic distinction, not just a matter of pallor brought about by seclusion, is suggested by, for example, the description of "white-armed" Nausicaa *outdoors* washing laundry and playing ball with her handmaidens.[54] Several scholars have suggested that the women of the *Iliad* and the *Odyssey* seem to have more freedom than later, more-documented women of Athens are said to have had in contemporary literary sources. The picture that emerges is a society in which some women, such as Calypso and Circe, seem to have a great deal of autonomy. However, they are foreigners, and while Penelope takes the initiative in trying to hold off the suitors, she cannot order them to leave and, without a male head of the house, is unable to ensure the well-being of her household.[55] A number of problems are inherent in using Homer for documentation, not the least of which is the debate over the date of the *Iliad* and *Odyssey* and the key corollary question—What society do these poems reflect?[56] We know that the

---

53. On the opening-up of Egypt to the Greeks, see J. Boardman, *The Greeks Overseas* (London: Thames and Hudson, 1980); W. Burkert, *The Orientalizing Revolution: Near Eastern Influence in the Early Archaic Age* (Cambridge: Harvard University Press, 1992), 14.

54. E. Irwin, *Colour Terms in Greek Poetry* (Toronto: Edgar Kent, 1974), 112.

55. S. Pomeroy, *Goddesses, Whores, Wives and Slaves: Women in Classical Antiquity* (New York: Schocken, 1975), 30; I. Morris, "Archaeology and Gender Ideologies in Early Archaic Greece," *Transactions of the American Philological Association* 129 (1999): 305. See also F. G. Naerebout, "Male-Female Relationships in the Homeric Epics," in *Sexual Asymmetry: Studies in Ancient Society*, ed. J. Blok and P. Mason (Amsterdam: J. C. Gieben, 1987), 109–46.

56. There is a huge bibliography on this topic. J. Hurwit, "Art Poetry and the Polis in the Age of Homer,"

Peisistratids commissioned a standardized performance of the poems in the late sixth century BC, which seems to have fixed the version current at that time as the canonical one. Yet the events described in the poems, the Trojan War and its aftermath, would have occurred (if they actually happened) during the Late Bronze Age, the world of the Mycenaeans. Indeed some of the objects described in the poems (boar's tusk helmets, for example) are characteristic Bronze Age artifacts. On the other hand, iron, the metal of the eighth century BC, is used by the Homeric protagonists. Yet the protagonists of the story are aristocrats, kings, and warriors, not citizens of a polis. Are we then dealing with the social mores of the Bronze Age, the eighth century, the archaic period, or a mixture of all of these? In addition, hovering over all of the discussion is the fact that, whatever the date(s), the poems were not designed to be a recitation of historical events. As Hurwit notes: "One of the ways in which 'Homeric society' does not correspond with any of the several ages through which the oral epic tradition passed is the absence of pottery, especially painted pottery, from its material culture."[57] The epics are thus not field reports from the past, but poetic evocations. What we admire so much in them—the artistry, the turns of phrase, the plots—are all infused with artistic license.

Hesiod also sounds themes with which male/female color differentiation is clearly compatible. He emphasizes that men and women are fundamentally different, indeed that they are different species. He is, after all, the source who tells of the creation of the first woman, "Pandora," establishing woman as not simply a different sex but a completely different kind of being. As Zeitlin has noted, this woman, unlike the biblical Eve, is not created to be a helpmeet for mankind but is rather a great evil that brings with her all of the other evils that will bedevil men.[58] Woman as evil or an uncontrollable force becomes a consistent trope in Greek literature. The added layer of differentiation, beyond the marker of secondary sexual characteristics or costume, which color provides strongly emphasizes this viewpoint. Hesiod also describes women as belonging to the interior of the house. While this might suggest that women are secluded, remember that this is where Hesiod *believes* women belong, not necessarily where they are in reality confined. Women had to at least leave the house to take part

in *From Pasture to Polis: Art in the Age of Homer*, ed. S. Langdon (Columbia, 1993), 14–42, provides a clear exposition of the problems.

57. J. Hurwit, "Art Poetry and the Polis in the Age of Homer," in S. Langdon, ed., *From Pasture to Polis: Art in the Age of Homer* (Columbia: University of Missouri Press, 1993), 29.

58. F. Zeitlin, *Playing the Other: Gender and Society in Classical Greek Literature* (Chicago: University of Chicago Press, 1996), 57.

in religious rituals if nothing else, although of course shopping, midwifery, visiting, fetching water, and so on would all have taken a woman outside the confines of the house. Hesiod, like Homer (remember Nausicaa, white-armed and outside), is making a distinction based on ideology—men belong to the outside and women to the inside. It is this claim that male/female color differentiation so emphatically marks. Women are fundamentally different from men, not only in their respective spheres of activity but also in their very nature, an alien race living in the midst of men. Shanks, for example, sees the subject matter of proto-Corinthian vase painting as asserting a world of elite men by showing their pre-occupations—warfare, hunting, and so on. Women are rarely shown.[59] He would also relate the animal friezes that are still very prevalent to a world of elite men, as female animals are rarely shown. Unlike in Athens, the human figure is not the major subject of vase decoration. Indeed, one of the reasons why Corinth is often considered to be more receptive to eastern influences is that it did not, like Athens, have a strong geometric figure tradition. The eastern animals resonate more strongly with Corinthian vase painters than does the human figure.

Thus it should not be surprising that when the Greeks encountered Egyptian art in which male and female were distinguished by color they would have incorporated this distinction into their own art. The artistic choice fits perfectly with their world view, even if it reflected a different cultural construct than that used by the Egyptians. We can see a slightly different borrowing in the Greek figure of the sphinx. The Egyptian prototype, a combination of pharaoh and a lion, is a positive icon of kingly power. The Greek version is also a power image, but a negative depiction of the monstrous power of evil embodied by woman. In the case of male/female color differentiation no change was necessary since the dark/light contrast fit so well with Greek ideas.

Ian Morris has suggested that sharp distinction between male and female also resonates with the political climate of the eighth century, which he sees as a struggle between two contesting ideologies. On one side are "elites," who promote an older way of doing things and what he calls a "middling" ideology of those more tied to the polis than to hereditary standards of prestige.[60] Certain

59. M. Shanks, "Art and Archaeology of Embodiment: Some Aspects of Archaic Greece," *Cambridge Archaeological Journal* 5, No. 2 (1999): 211.

60. I. Morris, *Archaeology as Cultural History: Words and Things in Iron Age Greece.* Contra see S. P. Morris, "Greek and Near Eastern Art in the Age of Homer," in S. Langdon, ed., *New Light on a Dark Age: Exploring the Culture of Geometric Greece*, 70–71.

aspects of male/female color differentiation dovetail nicely with this theory. The "middling" ideology stresses the unity of male citizens and thus marks clear distinctions between male and female. We can see this as well in a change in house layout from one room, the common form in earlier houses, to multi-room courtyard houses. The increase in rooms provides the opportunity for some separation of male and female, and the courtyard can serve as a means of restricting access to the interior.[61] On the other hand, Morris would link the aristocratic ethos with a more ideologically equal view of women as expressed in the poetry of Homer. Homer has clear elements of separation between the sexes in place as well. As mentioned above, he uses dark and light color imagery to describe men and women. He also uses light and dark to distinguish between correct and incorrect male behavior, with darkness being prized over (feminine?) lightness; the normal state of the inner man's emotions was characterized as dark, while an agitated state was described as light.[62]

Dean-Jones has noted that even death is divided along gender lines in the *Iliad* and the *Odyssey*.[63] Women are killed by Artemis and men by Apollo. While the Egyptian-style male/female color differentiation of the polychrome vases fits with his "middling" ideology that emphasizes sharp gender distinctions, it is also associated with aristocratic burials. Male/female color differentiation thus certainly resonates with ideas expressed in poets of the eighth century BC; it cannot, however, necessarily be clearly connected to a particular political viewpoint, although in Athens at least it does occur in connection with wealth.

Polychrome vase painting is a short-lived phenomenon. Because most of the vases come from a funerary context, they could represent a special type of production. Practical considerations may also be at work. Polychromy is better suited to wall painting (which although not preserved is mentioned in later authors as having been important again during this period) since many added colors could have been an extra step that slowed down the production process, at least in black figure, the presumed model for the other polychrome vases. Thus it became more economical to decrease the number of colors and thus the time it took to create a vase. In this vein Hurwit suggests that vase painters

61. I. Morris, "Archaeology and Gender Ideologies in Early Archaic Greece," 306. See also F. Lang, "Structural Change in Archaic Greek Housing," in *Ancient Greek Houses and Households*, ed. B. Ault and L. Nevett (Philadelphia: University of Pennsylvania Press, 2005), 12–35.

62. E. Irwin, *Colour Terms in Greek Poetry*, 113.

63. L. Dean-Jones, *Women's Bodies in Classical Greek Science* (Oxford: Oxford University Press, 1994), 111.

recognized that they could still be competitive in the marketplace if they offered less elaborately colored vases.[64]

The multi-color palette is reduced to black with reserved clay and added white and red. However, even within this limited palette, male/female color differentiation remains. The Egyptian brown/white distinction is replaced by black and white. When men and women are depicted, the men are the dark silhouette of black figure while the women are usually drawn in outline. Because Corinthian clay fires to a light, buff color, female skin is no longer indicated by an additional layer of white paint. This simplification of technique preserves an essential male/female difference while at the same time conforming to the streamlining of the production process that the move away from polychromy seems to represent. Yet for the Corinthian vase painter the connection of male flesh with red established in the Egyptian tradition remains strong. Male figures are sometimes shown with added red paint for faces and other areas of exposed flesh, as, for example, on a cup with *komast* dancers and a krater depicting Herakles banqueting with Iole.[65] Boardman suggests that this color indicates "a weather-beaten tan."[66] However, a connection to Egyptian practice is more probable than an explanation relying on an early use of "naturalism." Ideological distinction between male and female is the operative factor.

Athenian vase painters adopt the full black-figure technique by around 630 BC.[67] A transitional figure from Proto-Attic vase painting to fully realized black figure is the painter of Berlin A 34 (formerly known as the Woman Painter).[68] His earlier production is within the Proto-Attic tradition. Male and female are drawn in outline with added white paint for skin. The color scheme is thus restricted to black and white. On a later vase he paints the figure of a sphinx in black silhouette and overlays its face with white paint. Sphinxes are, of course, female in Greek art and mythology, so the use of white is appropriate. However, this sphinx representation is more complex than it appears at first glance. The black silhouette imitates Corinthian black figure, yet on Corinthian vases female faces are depicted in outline and left the buff color of the clay. Athenian

---

64. J. M. Hurwit, *The Art and Culture of Early Greece, 1100–480 BC*, 163.
65. Louvre E 635. J. Boardman, *Early Greek Vase Painting*, Fig. 396. 1, 2.
66. J. Boardman, *Athenian Black Figure Vases* (London: Thames and Hudson, 1974), 197.
67. On these vases see A. Alexandridou, *The Early Black-figured Pottery of Attika in Context (c. 630–570 BCE)* (Leiden: Brill, 2011).
68. Painter of Berlin A 34. J. Boardman, *Athenian Black Figure Vases*, 20. Crater Stand, Fig. 3 from Aegina, J. D. Beazley, *Attic Black-Figure Vase-Painters* (New York: Hacker Art Books, 1978), 1; Sphinx: Athens Kerameikos Museum 801, from Athens, ABV 1, 2.

clay has a much higher iron content than Corinthian and, consequently, fires to an orange color. If the Athenian artist had used the outline technique for this figure, the resulting skin tone of the unpainted face would have been orange rather than white, a color similar to the dark color sometimes used for female skin during the Amarna period, as on the bust of Nefertiti.[69]

Yet there may be something more to the use of white on this Athenian vase. The artist is, on the one hand, emulating the black-figure style of Corinth, but, on the other, is not keeping with Corinthian black-figure style in using white for a sphinx's face. The faces and chests of most Corinthian sphinxes, if painted, have added red paint.[70] This difference occurs despite the fact that during this period, as Alexandridou notes, there is a prominence of "Korinthianizing" characteristics in vase shapes.[71]

As mentioned above, red is also used for male faces in Corinthian black figure. Males and monstrous females are connected through this shared skin color, while other female figures are drawn in outline and retain the natural buff color of the fired clay. This can be seen on a cup by the Medallion painter.[72] On the exterior of the cup, sirens are solid black figure while the interior of the cup is decorated with a female face drawn in outline. Does the choice of male skin color for these female monsters suggest that their monstrous nature is a combination of male and female elements? The fact that the same use of red also holds true in Corinthian vase painting for another female composite figure—the siren—suggests that these monsters are a combination of male and female. However, there are also depictions of purely male sirens and sphinxes. Their masculine gender is indicated by beards. If these examples were earlier than the red-bodied female sirens and sphinxes, it would be possible to say that the masculine form was assimilated to a female version, with male skin color indicating a dual nature for the monster, but this is not the case. Bearded examples, although few, appear throughout the sixth century and are not confined to Corinth.[73]

What is noteworthy, though, is that Corinthian black-figure vase painters

69. On Attic clay see J. V. Noble, *Techniques of Painted Attic Pottery* (revised edition, London: Thames and Hudson, 1978), 21.

70. Among the many examples see an olpe by the Sphinx painter: NY 96.18.38, D. A. Amyx, *Corinthian Vase-painting of the Archaic Period* (Berkeley: University of California Press, 1988), 71–72 and pl. 24, 2a.

71. A. Alexandridou, *The Early Black-figured Pottery of Attika in Context (c. 630–570 BCE)*, 38.

72. Boston 12. 422: D. A. Amyx, *Corinthian Vase-painting of the Archaic Period*, 195 and Pl.76, 1a–c.

73. D. Tsiafakis, "ΠΕΛΩΡΑ: Fabulous Creatures and/or Demons of Death?" in *The Centaur's Smile: The Human Animal in Early Greek Art*, ed. J. M. Padgett (New Haven: Yale University Press, 2003), 73–104.

use red to depict the flesh of monstrous females, but not that of other women, while Attic vase painters emphasize the female gender of these beasts by painting them the same white color as other women. This distinction becomes firmer as Attic black figure develops. Corinthian black figure eventually adopts this color scheme, influenced by the dominance of Athenian vase painting. Added white is clearly used to mark sphinxes and sirens as well as other females on later Corinthian vases. There are, of course, exceptions. The "first recognizable artistic personality" among Attic black-figure vase painters[74]—the Nessos painter—does use red for some monster faces, but in general Attic vase painters follow the pattern described above. From their earliest imitation and eventual adoption of black-figure style, Athenian vase painters emphasize a clear male/female distinction through the use of added white even in areas where their Corinthian models do not.

The technique of added white paint over black-figure silhouette for female flesh used in the Athenian vase attributed to the painter of Berlin A 34 discussed above becomes the norm in fully developed Attic black figure, but is not always present in early works. Strong Corinthian influence is evident in the use of outline for female faces in the works of such early Attic black-figure painters as Sophilos.[75] His vases are decorated with rows of animals in the Corinthian style. The exposed flesh of women on his vases, although drawn in outline, is filled in with added white. The same can be said of one of the masterpieces of early black figure, the François vase signed by Kleitias (as painter) and Ergotimos (as potter) shown in Figure 17.[76] Many registers of the vase depict scenes associated with the life of Achilles. Goddesses and mortal women are all drawn in outline with added white paint, while the male figures are left in the dark black-figure silhouette. Since, as mentioned above, Athenian clay fires to an orange color rather than the buff of Corinthian, added white paint on women drawn in outline on Athenian vases further establishes light skin color, which was a given for figures drawn in outline on Corinthian vases.

Yet painting white over the fired clay does not seem to have provided enough contrast for Athenian vase painters. The work of some early Athenian cup painters, the so-called Siana cup painters (ca. 575–555 BC), brings to the

74. J. Boardman, *Athenian Black Figure Vases*, 15.

75. B. Cohen, "Outline in Black- and Red-Figure Vase-Painting: Outline as a Special Technique in Black- and Red-figure Vase-painting," in *The Colors of Clay*, ed. B. Cohen (Los Angeles: J. Paul Getty Museum, 2006), 152.

76. Florence Museum 4209, from Chiusi. J. D. Beazley, *Attic Black-Figure Vase-Painters*, 76, 1. J. Boardman, *Athenian Black Figure Vases*, Figs. 46 and 46.7.

fore what will be the more standard practice for indicating female flesh, namely, added white over the black-figure silhouette. In either case the added white paint tends to flake off, so paint adherence would not seem to be a technical consideration driving this choice.[77] It may be that it was "easier" to paint all of the silhouettes in one style and then differentiate with paint after firing.[78] The use of added white paint results in a very sharp and striking contrast between the black male figure and the white female.

While added red paint as well as added white is also used for details of clothing, furniture, and other features, white on top of black silhouette becomes the standard treatment for female flesh in Attic black-figure vase painting. Mortal and divine figures are both treated in this fashion. The reader need only recall a walk through any exhibit of Attic black-figure vases to confirm the ubiquity of white flesh for women and black for men. Seventh-century polychrome vases laid the groundwork for this development with their use of brown wash for male flesh. As we saw, Proto-Attic vase painters could use light color for men and women while also producing male figures with dark bodies and light faces. The sharp black/white contrast of Attic black figure is also not a direct inheritance from the Corinthian style of black figure, where outline is preferred for women and added red paint can also be used for males and monstrous women.

By the third quarter of the sixth century, Attic black figure becomes, as Proto-Corinthian vase painting had been during its heyday, the dominant vase-painting style in Greece and is widely imported and imitated. Sharp black/white differentiation of male and female by color is such standard practice on these vases that scholars have been lulled into thinking that this is simply convention with no underlying significance. Yet as the following survey of vases from other regions shows, even in imitations of Attic black figure male/female color differentiation is practiced with far less rigidity than it is in Athens, suggesting that there may be a special significance attached to the practice of gender-based color in Attic black figure.

77. Lip Cups: B. Cohen, "Outline in Black- and Red-Figure Vase-Painting: Outline as a Special Technique in Black- and Red-figure Vase-painting," in B. Cohen, *The Colors of Clay*, Nos. 41 and 42, 164–67. See also P. Heeson, *Athenian Little Master Cups* (Amsterdam: P. Heesen, 2011).

78. E. Aloupi-Siotis, "Discovery and Revival of Attic Vase Decoration Techniques: What Can They Offer Archaeological Research?" in *Papers on Special Techniques in Athenian Vases*, ed. K. Lapatin (Los Angeles: J. Paul Getty Museum 2008), 125, notes that Athenian potters did "adopt tricks of the trade" to "reduce unit cost by increasing production yield," although she does not specifically address added white paint.

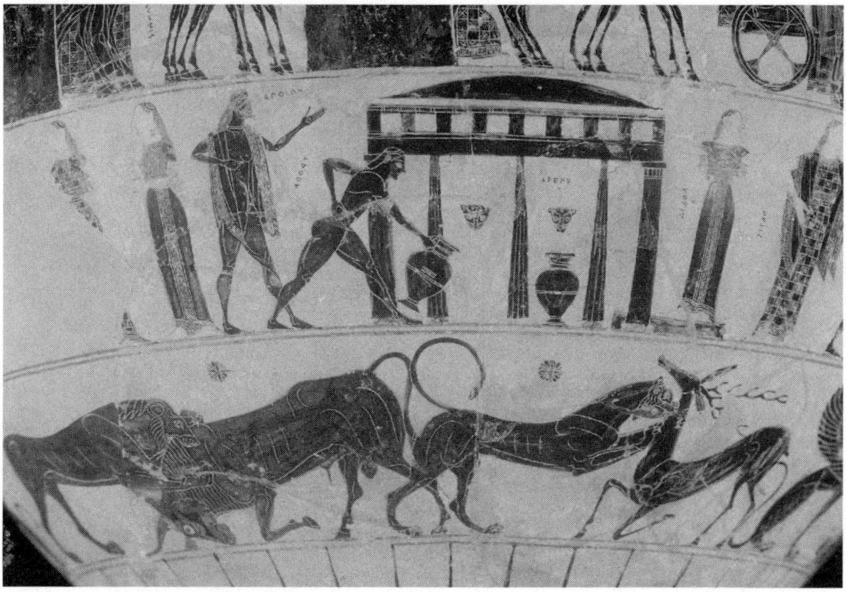

Fig. 17. Detail from the François vase. Kleitias (575–560 BC) and Ergotimos (potter, sixth century BC): scene and fighting animals. Attic black-figure volute crater, from Chiusi ca. 570 BC. (Museo Archeologico, Florence, Italy. Photo Credit: Scala/Art Resource, NY.)

In Corinth, for example, while vase painters imitate Athenian style by emphasizing mythological rather than animal scenes and paint their vases with a reddish-orange wash to give the appearance of Attic clay, they employ a more fluid use of color than their Attic black-figure models. One vase in particular, an amphora by the Tydeus Painter (Fig. 18), has received considerable attention for its use of white paint for male flesh.[79] The vase shows a nude male, Tydeus, painted in black-figure silhouette, threatening with a sword Ismene, who reclines on a couch. Ismene's exposed flesh (her upper body from below the breasts) is painted white. Running from the scene is a nude white-painted male identified by inscription as her lover, Theoclymenos. The use of white for the escaping lover has caused numerous scholars to suggest that the artist is using

79. Louvre E 640, D. A. Amyx, *Corinthian Vase-painting of the Archaic Period*, No. 6, 393, 270.

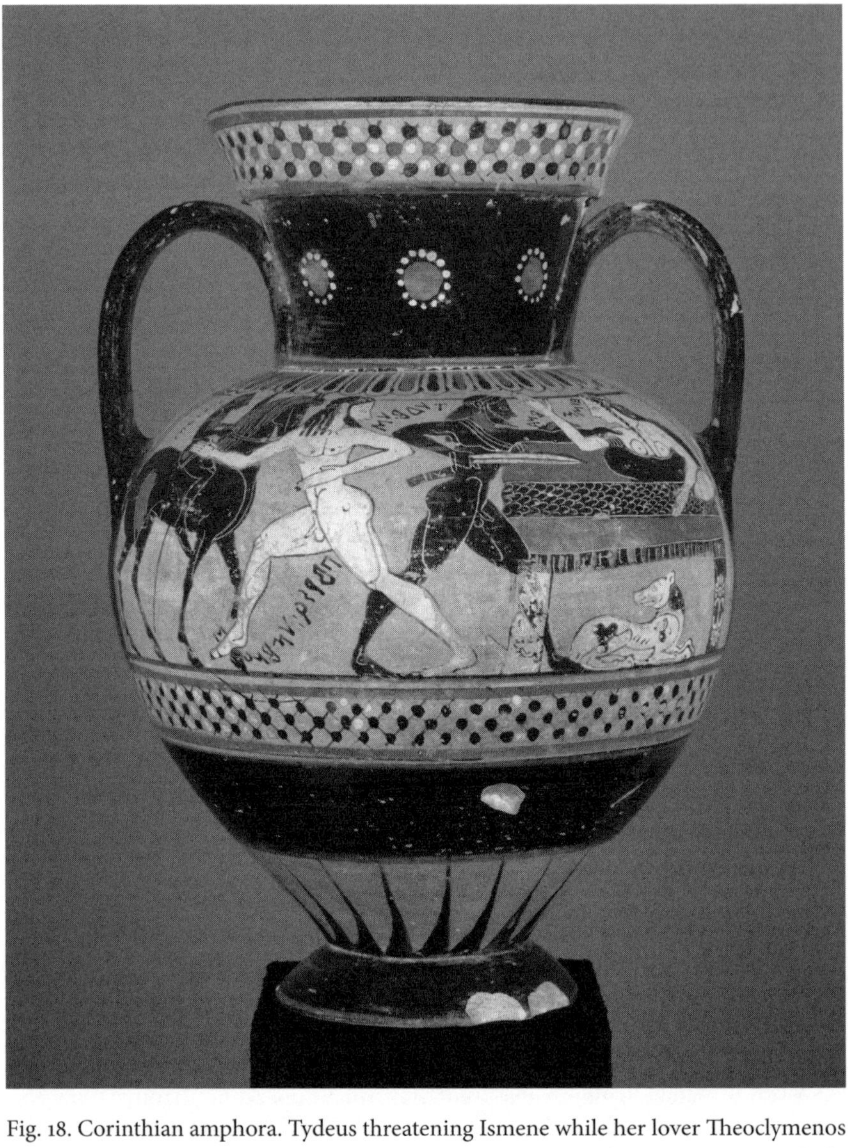

Fig. 18. Corinthian amphora. Tydeus threatening Ismene while her lover Theoclymenos escapes. Late style I, ca. 570–560 BC. H. 32 cm. Inv.: E 640. (Photo: Hervé Lewandoski Louvre, Paris, France. Photo Credit: Réunion des Musées Nationaux/Art Resource, NY.)

color to indicate a cowardly male.[80] Yet this argument is based on universalizing the Athenian black-male/white-female approach to color.

If we look at more than just this vase, we see that in Corinthian vase painting the Attic color convention is not as strictly adhered to. White is used to create a coloristic effect and to form a sharp contrast, not so much with the black as with the red background surface with which Corinthian vases are now being painted.[81] We can see an early example of this in a vase dated to "before the mid sixth century" in Copenhagen.[82] On one side warriors are grouped in combatant pairs with a fallen warrior at the feet of each pair. The figures are labeled, but no specific mythological scene has been identified. The combatants are painted in standard black-figure silhouette. The fallen warrior at the feet of the pair on the left is, however, painted white. At first glance this might suggest that white is used to show defeat and that is the loser is "feminized." Yet in the other pair the vanquished is also painted in black-figure silhouette with no added white paint. Rather than being strictly a gender indicator, white is used throughout the surface of this vase to provide a visual contrast. Thus in Pair One, the right combatant has a shield crest painted in white that balances the white paint of the shield of his opponent. In Pair Two, the shield crest and chest armor of the left combatant is painted white. His opponent's shield is decorated with a white-painted Gorgon shield device. The black-silhouetted dying figure at their feet has a shield painted with alternating black and white pinwheels. The overall decorative pattern is one of balanced contrasts set up by the use of added white paint. Thus white, in this case, is used for coloristic effect. The white body of the "cowardly" lover on the Tydeus Painter's vase provides just such a color contrast. He is positioned between a dark-silhouetted male chariot driver and the dark silhouette of Tydeus. We have an alteration of dark and light culminating in the white body of Ismene. Tydeus' leg is contrasted against a white painted leg of the couch on which Ismene reclines, and a white dog is painted under the couch.

This employment of added white paint is seen in another one of this painter's vases in which a siren stands between two sphinxes. In this case the flesh color of the monstrous females follows Attic convention; it is painted white. But

80. J. Henderson, "Smashing Bodies: The Corinthian Tydeus and Ismene Amphora (Louvre E 640)," in *Constructions of the Classical Body*, ed. J. I. Porter (Ann Arbor: University of Michigan Press, 1999), 19–49.

81. D. A. Amyx, *Corinthian Vase-painting of the Archaic Period*, 393.

82. Copenhagen NM 13531: J. Boardman, *The History of Greek Vases: Potters, Painters and Pictures* (London: Thames and Hudson, 2001), Fig. 55.

the females are also part of the Corinthian love of polychromy. Not just the faces of the figures are painted white, as they would be in Attic vase painting, but also their entire bodies, with the exception of the wings. This creates a contrast of large areas of white with the orange wash of the clay. Indeed Rasmussen has suggested that rather than competition with Athenian vases the aesthetic possibilities of this type of contrast may even have been the impetus for the Corinthian adoption of orange wash for their vases during this period.[83] Colorful effect predominates over the sharp male/female color differentiation of Athenian vases.

In East Greek vases we also see that the sharp color/gender distinctions of Attic vases do not hold true. "East Greece" is a catchall name for the location of a number of these vase-painting styles, although a specific city of origin cannot always be pinned down. Among these productions Caeretan hydriae stand out.[84] Their figure style is very similar to East Greek (Ionian sculpture), and the subject matter betrays a detailed grasp of Greek mythology. Strikingly and significantly for our investigation, these hydriae do not follow Attic color and gender conventions. Male skin can be black, but also white and red. The skin of women is white, although on one vase Leto and Artemis are both painted red.[85] While, as discussed above, some have argued, as in the case of the Corinthian Tydeus amphora, for the use of white on male flesh as an indication of cowardice, no such connection can be made for the use of white on these vases. In Figure 19, the strongest and bravest of Greek heroes, Herakles, appears with white skin. A white Herakles brings the monstrous three-headed hound of Hades, Cerberus, to a terrified and also white-painted Eurystheus on another hydria.[86] The god Hephaestos is painted white on a hydria with scenes of the god in the presence of satyrs and maenads.[87] If all male figures were white, one could connect the practice to the Assyrian color system. If only certain types of male figures were painted white, one could also look for iconographic significance, but this is not the case. Like Corinthian vases, Caeretan hydriae have

83. T. Rasmussen, "Corinth and Orientalizing," in *Looking at Greek Vases*, ed. T. Rasmussen and N. Spivey (Cambridge: Cambridge University Press, 1991), 76.

84. This group of vases has a limited production and was found primarily in Etruscan tombs. The major study is J. M. Hemelrijk, *Caeretan Hydriae* (Mainz am Rhein: Zabern, 1984).

85. Male skin: J. M. Hemelrijk, *Caeretan Hydriae*. 1: London BM 188.7–25/30; 12: Louvre Campana 10.227, and 35 Leipzig Coll T 3337 (now lost); Leto and Artemis, No. 12 p.57 c-d.

86. Louvre E 701. J. M. Hemelrijk, *Caeretan Hydriae*, No. 4, p. 14 pl. 32.

87. Vienna Kunsthistorisches Museum 3577, J. M. Hemelrijk, *Caeretan Hydriae*, No. 5, pp.14–15 pl. 36.

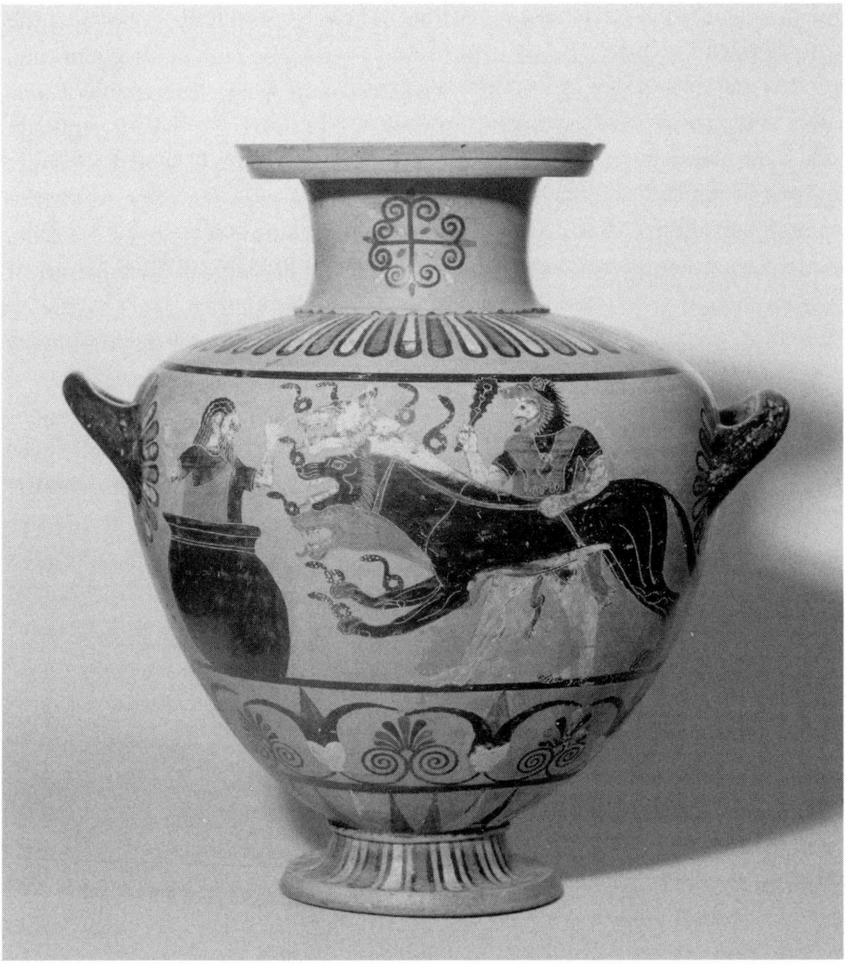

Fig. 19. Side A of a black figure hydria. Herakles leading Cerberus to Eurystheus. From Cerveteri. Ca. 525 BC. Inv.: E 701. (Photo: Hervé Lewandowski. Louvre, Paris, France. Photo Credit: Réunion des Musées Nationaux/Art Resource, NY.)

much added white for details other than skin color. Floral decoration, armor, furniture, and such are also painted white.

The main scene of a hydria decorated with a scene of Herakles and the pharaoh Bousiris reveals a complex combination of gender symbolism, coloristic effect, and Near Eastern influence.[88] According to the myth, Bousiris, king of Egypt and son of Poseidon, had been instructed by a seer to sacrifice a foreigner to maintain the fruitfulness of his kingdom. The king zealously adopted this practice after first sacrificing the seer and then all foreigners. Herakles, on his way to obtain the Apples of the Hesperides, was captured by the king and, although he allowed himself to be led to the sacrificial altar, soon overcame his captors and killed Bousiris and all of his sons.

On the hydria, a nude, bearded Herakles flings his captors, much smaller robed priests, in a variety of directions as they try to move him toward the altar for the sacrifice. The scene bears a striking resemblance to Egyptian images of pharaoh smiting his enemies. In these scenes, Herakles, just as pharaoh, is portrayed as much larger than his victims. The scene plays with the traditional iconography by casting Herakles in the role of smiter, while the Egyptians are victims.[89] Another factor in this play on Egyptian tradition, one that has been largely overlooked by scholars, is that Herakles is painted red. As we have seen in Chapters 1 and 2, red is the standard color that signifies the Egyptian male. In depictions of the peoples of the world, Egyptian artists use yellow and black for other ethnicities, but their own men are red. On the hydria the priests with whom Herakles grapples are painted with either a yellowish cream-colored skin or they are black-figure silhouette. One could associate the yellowish cream color with the color used for female skin. However, in this instance the use of this particular shade rather than simply white is also linked to the fact that the garments of the priests are painted white and the skin thus contrasts with the garments. The white garments are a feature that adds to the Egyptian setting of the scene, as they are a typical Egyptian priestly costume.

The light-skinned male priests are not behaving in any less heroic fashion than those who are left in black-figure silhouette. That is, the dark figures are not prevailing. Rather, the figures, with the exception of two light figures at the feet of Herakles, alternate dark and light. This is a principle we have also seen in

88. Vienna Kunsthistorisches Museum 3576, J. M. Hemelrijk, *Caeretan Hydriae*, No. 34, pp. 50–51, pl. 119.

89. M. C. Miller, "Myth of Bousiris," in *Not the Classical Ideal: Athens and the Construction of the Other in Greek Art*, ed. B. Cohen (Leiden: Brill Academic Publishers, 2000), 414.

Egyptian art, where overlapping figures in groups are painted in lighter shades of the same color. In the case of our vase, the figures do not overlap as tightly as in Egyptian scenes that make use of such a light/dark color alternation; rather, they more closely resemble the alternating dark and light figures in the admittedly much earlier (second millennium) Investiture fresco from the Palace of King Zimri-Limat Mari.

The use of contrasting figures continues on the neck of the hydria, which shows a boar hunt in which white-fleshed male hunters alternate with black-silhouette male hunters. The contrast is further emphasized by the fact that the white hunters wear dark costumes (black-figure silhouette) and the dark hunters wear white (added paint) costumes. This suggests to me that the use of red for Herakles is not simply a coloristic effect. Used in combination with the smiting pose, it clearly speaks of Egyptian art and plays with the Egyptian male superiority usually represented by that color. The alternating hunters and priests exhibit a similar familiarity with Egyptian use of contrast and also, perhaps, a desire for overall visual effects we saw in Corinthian vases of this period. Awareness of the Egyptian idea of displaying different peoples of the world with different skin colors, discussed in Chapter 1, is also present. Three skin colors are depicted—red, yellow, and black.

While visual contrast is emphasized in the use of two colors for the skin of the priests, the introduction of yellow also marks the Egyptians as ethnically distinct from Herakles. Under the hydria's handles are a group of figures painted in dark silhouette, further characterized, in the Egyptian style, as Nubians by their hair, weaponry, and facial features. The Bousiris hydria's color scheme thus shows a number of influences for the use of color on the same vase—Egyptian, Near Eastern, possibly Corinthian. This vase reveals the artist's very sophisticated understanding of Egyptian practice. Such familiarity does not necessarily mean that the artist had to see Egyptian monuments first hand, although some scholars have concluded that Caeretan vase painters were Ionian artists active in Etruria who spent time in Egypt.[90] Although the vase can be appreciated for its coloristic effects without understanding the parody of Egyptian practice, one wonders if the tweaking of Egyptian artistic forms presupposes an equally sophisticated audience.

Not all of the Caeretan hydriae display such a sophisticated use of color, but

90. Miller, "Myth of Bousiris," in B. Cohen, ed., *Not the Classical Ideal: Athens and the Construction of the Other in Greek Art*, 414.

what they do not display is the rigidity of skin color depiction characteristic of Attic vase painting. By comparing the Bousiris hydria with an Attic black-figure version of the same scene, we see this clearly. On a black-figure amphora of Type B attributed to the Swing painter and dated to ca. 540,[91] Herakles is shown fighting Egyptian priests at an altar, yet the scene does not have the clear dependence on Egyptian prototypes that the hydria showed. Herakles is the same size as his opponents. The composition with one figure draped over the altar is much more similar to images of the death of Priam at Troy than to pharaoh smiting his enemies.[92] White is used only for the robes of two of the priests, and all male figures are painted in the regular dark-silhouette technique of black figure. Clazomenian and Chiot wares as well often show white males.[93] While women are rare on Fikellura ware, they are treated with the same dark flesh as males.[94] Against the background of other wares, standard Athenian practice stands out.

There are, however, a few Athenian exceptions to the standard practice of added white over black silhouette for exposed female flesh. First are lip cups (so-named because the lip, the upper edge of the cup, is offset from the body and is not glazed), the majority of which date to the mid-sixth century.[95] Figure 20 is an example. Such vases are usually decorated with scenes in black-figure silhouette, but several painters create versions in which the lip is decorated with an image of the profile head of a woman drawn in outline, with no added white. The women on these so-called head cups wear jewelry, and their hair is bound either with a headcloth (*sakkos*) or an incised headband. For these cups, connection to a popular type of Corinthian representation may explain the use of outline and lack of color conformity. Such profile heads appear also on Corinthian round aryballoi[96] and on the interior of Corinthian cups. The fact that the image on one of the aryballoi is inscribed with a female name and the body of

---

91. Cincinnati Art Museum, purchase 1959. J. D. Beazley, *Paralipomena: Additions to Attic Black-figure Vase-painters and to Attic Red-figure Vase-painters*, second edition (Oxford: Oxford University Press, 1971), 134–23; J. Boardman, *Athenian Black Figure Vases*, Fig. 143; M. C. Miller, "Myth of Bousiris," in B. Cohen, ed., *Not the Classical Ideal: Athens and the Construction of the Other in Greek Art*, Fig. 16.3.
92. M. C. Miller, "Myth of Bousiris," in B. Cohen, ed., *Not the Classical Ideal: Athens and the Construction of the Other in Greek Art*, 413–42.
93. R. M. Cook, "A List of Clazomenian Pottery," *Annual of the British School at Athens*, Vol. 47 (1952): 147.
94. R. M. Cook, "Fikellura Pottery," *Annual of the British School at Athens*, Vol. 34 (1933/34): 68.
95. Lip Cups: B. Cohen, "Outline in Black- and Red-Figure Vase-Painting: Outline as a Special Technique in Black- and Red-figure Vase-painting" in B. Cohen, *The Colors of Clay*, 153.
96. H. Payne, *Necrocorinthia: A Study of Corinthian Art in the Archaic Period* (Oxford: Clarendon Press, 1931), 162; B. Cohen, *The Colors of Clay*.

the same vase with a list of male names has suggested an identification of these female heads as hetairai (prostitutes),[97] primarily because their names are given, which Classical literary sources suggest is inappropriate for "respectable" women. One could thus see the outline female heads as a device for indicating "women of ill-repute." (We will have more to say about this in Chapter 4.) However, the fact that the goddess Athena is also drawn in outline on a lip cup attributed to the Epitimos Painter[98] militates against identifying outline as a technique reserved for hetairai. The fact that on the opposite side of the same cup the head of a male warrior is also drawn in profile might suggest that this particular cup is also too different from the standard treatment for males to be a criterion by which to judge whether the use of outline for female flesh is significant. But there are other examples of goddesses drawn in outline. Lydos, a highly skilled vase painter who flourished from ca. 560 to 540 BC, used outline for Athena, who fights alongside Herakles, on an oinochoe (jug) in Berlin.[99]

Outline images of the gorgoneion, the frontal face of the monstrous female gorgon Medusa (distinct from the running full-figured Gorgon, which is given the standard treatment), can also be attributed to Corinthian influence and provide another category of exceptions to the standard practice of using black silhouette with an overlay of white paint for females.[100] While frontal faces are unusual in early Greek vase painting, the staring face of the Gorgon emphasizes the power of her gaze to turn men to stone. In this case, however, the use of outline style on early Athenian vases is explained by the Corinthian origin of the gorgoneion, which was determined by Payne.[101] Thus for all of the vases discussed above, imitation of Corinthian practice could be an explanation for the use of the unpainted female outline face. This seems to hold particularly true for the Gorgon, since the representational type was invented in Corinth.

Another group, occurring in the work of the Amasis Painter whose career spans ca. 560 to 525 BC, is more intriguing. His use of outline for female figures

---

97. H. Payne, *Necrocorinthia*, 162; B. Cohen, "Outline in Black- and Red-Figure Vase-Painting: Outline as a Special Technique in Black- and Red-figure Vase-painting," in Cohen, *The Colors of Clay*, 152 Note 94. Contra see S. Lewis, *The Athenian Woman: An Iconographic Handbook* (London: Routledge, 2002), 107.
98. Copenhagen National Museum 13966, J. D. Beazley, Para 48, Cohen, "Outline in Black- and Red-Figure Vase-Painting: Outline as a Special Technique in Black- and Red-figure Vase-painting," in B. Cohen, *The Colors of Clay*, No. 41.
99. Oinochoe, Berlin Staatliche Museen 1732, ABV 110, 37. J. Boardman, *Attic Black Figure Vases*, Fig. 68.
100. H. Payne, *Necrocorinthia*, 86–87.
101. Ibid., 86–87.

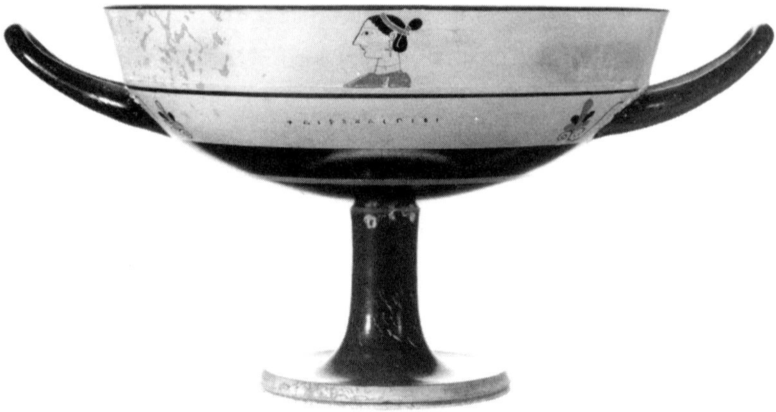

Fig. 20. Lip cup (kylix). The Sakonides Painter. Greek, Archaic Period, about 550–530 BC. Place of manufacture: Greece, Attica, Athens. Ceramic, black figure. Height 6 1/16 in (15.4 cm); diameter: 9 in (22.8 cm). (Museum of Fine Arts, Boston, Frederick Brown Fund, 66.816.)

on some of his vases has long been noted by scholars, who have variously identified it as a Corinthian trait or an early experiment with color that anticipates red figure.[102] The connection to Corinth is weakened by the fact that rather than appearing on vases dated early in his career, outline women occur on those from the middle years. Also, in the second quarter of the sixth century, Corinthian vase painters themselves are more closely imitating Attic painters by painting their clay with a red wash, and while still drawing many female figures in outline they are adding white paint.

Mertens notes in her study of the Amasis Painter vases, on which female figures are drawn in outline without added white paint, that such figures are limited to a mere half dozen vases, but that in all but one case they are depictions of maenads. She identifies the one exception as Thetis handing armor to her son Achilles. For Mertens this limited use of outline carries a specific meaning. As she states:

102. D. von Bothmer, *The Amasis Painter and His World: Vase-painting in Sixth-century B.C. Athens* (New York: Thames and Hudson, 1985). B. Cohen, "Outline in Black- and Red-Figure Vase-Painting: Outline as a Special Technique in Black- and Red-figure Vase-painting," in B. Cohen, ed., *The Colors of Clay*, 154.

> They (the maenads), like the shield bearer (Thetis), were beings whom no one had really seen or studied, so that in depicting them, the Amasis Painter could allow his creative imagination some latitude. He was not bound to render what everyone could observe, and he did not have to be totally "orthodox" in using standard black-figure. What he developed was an idiom that allowed him to depict and characterize these invisible presences while, at the same time, maintaining the clarity and precision of his presentation. [103]

I cannot agree with her assertion that these images represent beings "no one had really seen" since that observation could apply to any of the many mythological figures in the Greek world. However, I do like her observation that, in these instances, the Amasis Painter confines this technique to specific types of female figures, those that are neither goddess nor mortal.

The Amasis Painter's use of outline for maenads could be an expression of the maenads' licentiousness. They are free to roam the woods with the Dionysos and engage in acts of sexual abandon beyond the norms of the typical woman. However, as Mertens points out, the painter's use of outline is primarily limited to these types of figures. He does not experiment with his male figures in this way. While some have seen his use of outline as the first step to red figure, it is important to note that, as witnessed by its use in Corinthian vases, outline is an old technique. Red figure is not an outline style but rather the reverse silhouette style of black figure.[104]

Still one cannot totally rule out the possibility that the Amasis Painter is experimenting with outline for artistic effect and not in an iconographically significant way. Despite the painter's use of outline for some females, the fact that the males in these scenes are painted in black-figure silhouette means that a dark male/light female contrast is still at work. He may have tried to use outline to distinguish between overlapping figures as, for example, on a vase in Paris[105] where two maenads drape their arms around each other. The arms of each are clearly outlined. However, clarity is not gained since it is very difficult to tell which arm belongs to which figure. The figures are in fact much clearer

---

103. J. R. Mertens, "The Amasis Painter: Artist and Tradition," in K. Lapatin, ed., *Getty Museum Papers on the Amasis Painter and His World* (Malibu: Getty Museum, 1997). maenads: 171, 175.
104. B. Cohen, "Outline in Black- and Red-Figure Vase-Painting: Outline as a Special Technique in Black- and Red-figure Vase-painting," in B. Cohen, ed., *The Colors of Clay*, 154.
105. Neck Amphora, Paris Bibliotheque Nationale, Cabinet des Médailles 222; J. D. Beazley, *Attic Black-Figure Vase-Painters*, 152, No. 25 Side B: D. von Bothmer, *The Amasis Painter and His World*, No. 23, 125–29, Detail 126.

on an amphora, also in Paris,[106] in which he paints the maenads in the traditional white-over-black technique. The fact that he does not use outline for every maenad—figures on subsidiary friezes, even on vases where the main scene is done in outline, are painted in the traditional black figure with added white paint—could also support the idea that he is simply experimenting, although again the fact that he is primarily using outline on a specific type of figure argues against this. The Amasis Painter uses added red for the flesh of two figures of Athena.[107] This color is often used by Corinthian vase painters for male figures. We may pertinently ask—Is he emphasizing Athena's somewhat dual nature as a warrior and a woman?

While the jury may still be out on the Amasis Painter's use of color as a message-bearing tool, a stronger case, I think, can be made for the use of color for the monstrous figures. In Attic vase painting, the gorgoneion is treated in outline, presumably because this image was created in Corinth, and the Athenians remain true to the original. Why then the emphasis on white skin for the other monstrous females? Attic vase painters want to make particularly clear the female nature of these creatures, the fact that woman can be monstrous. Clear demarcation between male and female through color becomes the hallmark of Attic vase painting, much more so than in Corinthian. As we shall see, for Athenians male/female color differentiation is a much more important distinction than elsewhere. Perhaps Pliny (NH. 35.55–56) recalls a distant memory of the Attic emphasis on this feature when he says that the first artist to distinguish between men and women in painting was an Athenian.

Even though Attic black figure dominates the market, local variants of black figure do not always adopt such a close adherence to Attic color conventions, suggesting that the Athenian color choice relates specifically to Athenian societal ideas and needs. Why is this differentiation so important to Athenians? It would, of course, be helpful if I could flip the question and answer why others did not find it so important, but our source material is so much more abundant

---

106. Panel Amphora (Type B), Paris Musée du Louvre: F3 (LP 2021; N 3502), J. D. Beazley, *Attic Black-Figure Vase-Painters* (Oxford, 1956), No. 6, 150; D. von Bothmer, *The Amasis Painter and His World*, No. 5, 51–83.

107. Fragmentary olpe, Oxford, Ashmolean Museum of Art and Archaeology, 1929, 19. D. Beazley, *Attic Black-Figure Vase-Painters*, No. 38, 153; D. von Bothmer, *The Amasis Painter and His World*, No. 29, 145–46; Oinochoe (Shape III: Chous) Paris Musée du Louvre F 37 (Cp 3237). D. Beazley, *Attic Black-Figure Vase-Painters*, No. 46, 154; D. von Bothmer, *The Amasis Painter and His World*, 156–58, Detail 156.

for Athens than for anywhere else that the best hope for an answer comes from framing the question with an Atheno-centric focus.

Remember, the first choice among scholars has been that this color convention represents a natural distinction between the outdoor lives of men and the indoor lives of women. As Boardman states about Attic black figure, "In black-figure women's flesh is painted white, but the men's left natural."[108] To reevaluate the commonly accepted "naturalness" of the dark/light color distinction between men and women in Athenian black figure, we need to look at many of the factors we explored in our examination of Egyptian color practices. First and foremost we might ask whether Athenian art of the Archaic period is given to naturalism. Elsewhere Boardman himself states that male/female color differentiation is the "only natural feature in an otherwise unrealistic art." As Hurwit states, "The shapes, postures, movements and gestures of Archaic figures are limited and typical and so are the situations in which they find themselves; the Archaic artist in other words generalizes"[109] as the following short list of stylized depictions in Archaic art indicates: (1) Running, for example, is depicted by the *knielauf* pose, in which a figure has a frontal torso and widespread profile legs with both knees touching the ground. (2) The complete eye is always shown even when the rest of the face is in profile. (3) Foreshortening is not used. (4) The only facial indication of emotion is the occasional portrayal of a figure with an open mouth.[110] Thus, added red for male flesh is a marker of *ideal* masculinity, not *real* sun exposure.

Of course, color is not the only feature that differentiates male from female. Costume and secondary sexual characteristics are depicted. Mature men wear beards, and the genitals of nude males are another obvious sign of masculinity (females are seldom shown nude during this period). There are other distinctions, perhaps less obvious to the modern viewer. McNiven has shown that even gestures were gender specific on Attic black- and red-figure vases.[111] Women are generally characterized by gestures that indicate emotion or lack of self-control. In funerary scenes, for example, men stand in ordered rows with their hands extended in identical position, which McNiven suggests is a formal

108. J. Boardman, *Pre-Classical: From Crete to Archaic Greece* (Baltimore: Penguin, 1997), 113.
109. J. M. Hurwit, *The Art and Culture of Early Greece*, 18.
110. On the open mouth, see J. Boardman, *Early Greek Vase Painting*, 266.
111. T. J. McNiven, "Behaving Like an Other: Telltale Gestures in Athenian Vase-Painting," in B. Cohen, ed., *Not the Classical Ideal*, 71–97.

dirge performed for the deceased, as opposed to the more-emotional and less-structured mourning of women, who instead exhibit a variety of arm positions, including tearing at their hair.[112] Acts of supplication, indicated by touching someone's chin, are usually made by women and are admissions of powerlessness.[113] Beginning in the first quarter of the sixth century BC, many scenes on Attic vases feature framing or "spectator" figures—men and women who stand on either side of the main scene and who observe the action. In a statistical study of such figures, Stansbury-O'Donnell identified gender-linked patterns of representation. Specifically, women are "more reactive than inert." For example, they raise their arms in alarm rather than quietly observing as do their male counterparts.[114] In a sense this could be a "realistic" way of depicting norms of social behavior and defining the accepted parameters of expression permissible to each group.

Boardman observed that "women's eyes are usually almond shaped, not the male saucers, and often have red pupils."[115] A less open gaze could connect to the reactive and less-initiatory roles for women on Greek vases. This would be a symbolic rather than an actual (realistic) difference, since it is unlikely that within the same population all of the women would have almond-shaped eyes and all of the men round ones.

Equally puzzling as far as "realism" is the presence of white-skinned females in outdoor settings as we see in Figure 21. Many of Stansbury-O'Donnell's female spectators are viewing events that could only have taken place outdoors. Indeed, many scenes involving women on Attic black-figure vases presuppose an outdoor setting, for example a scene of women swimming in a pond.[116] Yet the idea that women are pale because of actual female seclusion has been a difficult one to put to rest, especially because of the insistence of later predominantly Athenian Classical literary sources that this was practiced.[117] In particu-

112. Ibid., 72.

113. Ibid., 77.

114. M. Stansbury-O'Donnell, *Vase Painting, Gender and Social Identity in Archaic Athens* (Cambridge: Cambridge University Press, 2006), 232.

115. J. Boardman, *Athenian Black Figure Vases*, 198.

116. Rome Villa Giulia 2609, D. Beazley, *Paralipomena*, second edition, 1468 ter. See C. Bérard, "The Order of Women," in *A City of Images: Iconography and Society in Ancient Greece*, ed. C. Bérard, C. Bron, J-L. Durand, F. Frontisi-Ducroux, A. Lissarrague, A. Schnapp, and J. P. Vernant (Princeton: Princeton University Press, 1989), Fig. 128, 94.

117. For a history of the concept of female seclusion in the ancient Greek world, see H. S. Nielsen, "Women in Classical Athens—Their Social Space: Ideal and Reality," in *Sex and Difference in Ancient Greece and Rome*, ed. M. Golden and P. Toohey (Edinburgh: Edinburgh University Press, 2003), 23–30.

lar, in legal cases a description of the layout of the house prominently specifies separate quarters for men and women.[118] Other Classical sources such as Xenophon and Lysias describe houses that are physically separated into men's and women's quarters, which, as Nevett points out, has led to the modern belief that ancient Greek women were kept in seclusion.[119] I shall have more to say about Classical house design and seclusion in the next chapter. However, earlier houses have a much more restricted number of rooms, which allows for even less separation between household members. Indeed, as Nevett notes:

> Rather than secluding women within particular rooms of the house, this isolation was achieved by providing facilities specifically for male guests. The *gunaikon* presumably refers to the family area of the house, which those guests did not customarily enter.[120]

Thus both literature and actual remains of houses point to gender as an important principle ordering the arrangement of domestic space; rather than indicating seclusion, they suggest separation. Women's lighter skin does not reflect an actual seclusion, but rather an ideological seclusion. It provides an extra layer of differentiation between men and women and is a shorthand for the contrast in societal roles of the sexes.

We have seen that the idea that men and women are fundamentally different was given a mythological basis in the story of Pandora as related by Hesiod. In the sixth century, Ionian philosophers offer a physiological twist. Male and female bodies are, according to them, formed from different substances; men are solid and women are porous and spongy.[121] Black figure supports this ideology as well.

While the color symbolism of Egyptian sculpture and painting has long been recognized, fewer scholars have examined Archaic Greek art from this point of view. Two scholars who have attempted to systematize Archaic color use based on the extant artistic remains have reached quite different conclusions. Manzelli suggests that specific colors used by the Greeks on sculpture

118. J. Gould, "Law, Custom and Myth: Aspects of the Social Position of Women in Classical Athens," *Journal of Hellenic Studies* (1980): 38–59.
119. L. Nevett, *House and Society in the Ancient Greek World* (Cambridge: Cambridge University Press, 1999), 17.
120. Ibid., 154.
121. See L. Dean-Jones, "Women's Bodies in Classical Greek Science," in M. Golden and P. Toohey, eds., *Sex and Difference in Ancient Greece and Rome*, 184.

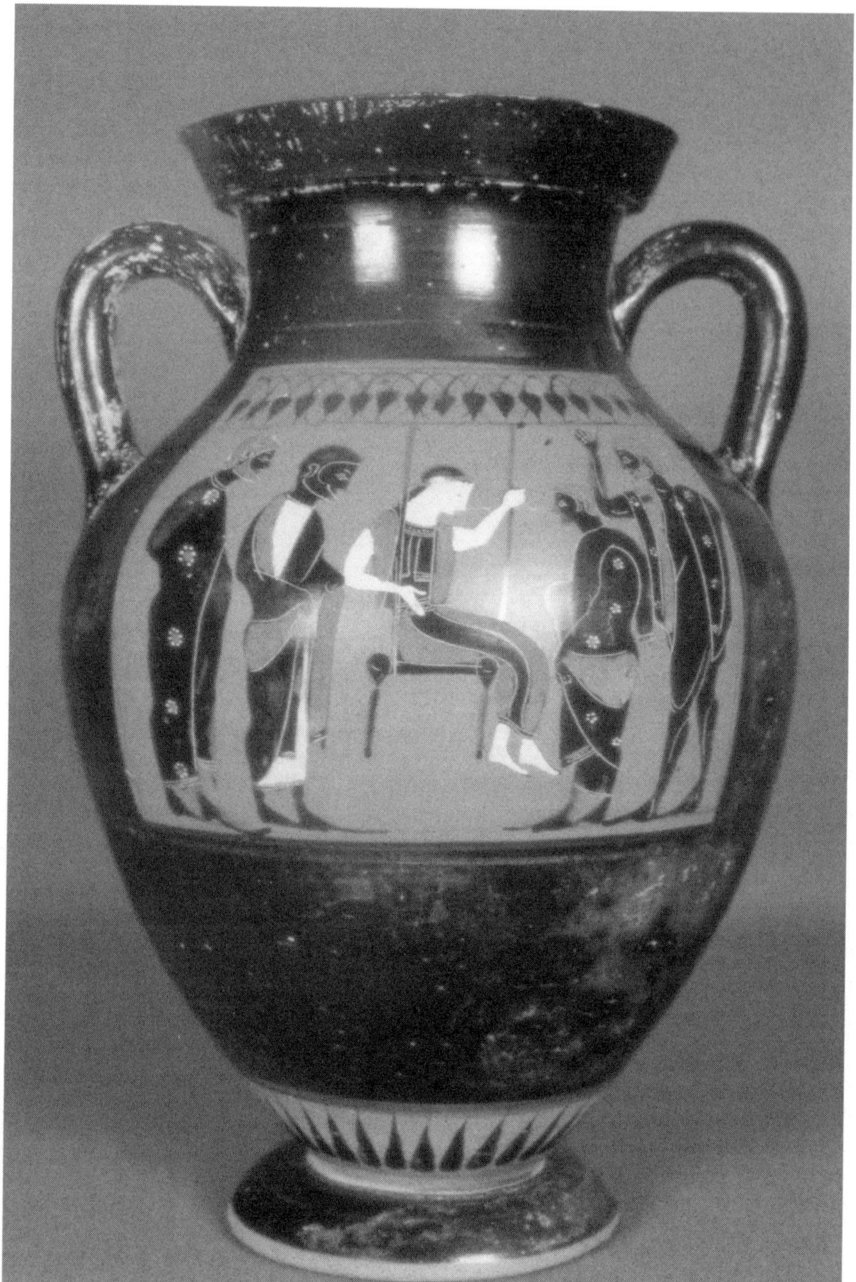

Fig. 21. Two-handled jar (amphora) depicting a woman in a swing and four men. The Swing Painter. Greek, Archaic Period, about 540–520 BC. Place of manufacture: Greece, Attica, Athens. Ceramic, black figure. Height 15 13/16 in (40.1 cm). (Museum of Fine Arts, Boston, Henry Lillie Pierce Fund, 98.918.)

carry symbolic meaning.[122] She connects red with blood and chthonic deities, but Greek literature does not consistently describe blood as red. Red as a background color is used not only on Archaic funerary monuments but also on temple pediments, yet Manzelli bases her connections on a belief that Indo-European languages share a common color system. This flies against most studies that show that color naming is very much a culture-specific phenomenon, not a broadly based characteristic. As Gage notes, "colour, in spite of widespread belief in the universality of certain colour-ideas, is like all formal characteristics ideologically neutral. It can be seen to have served a very wide range of aesthetic and symbolic purposes."[123] Walter-Karydi comes closer to the theoretical underpinnings of early Greek color in her analysis of vase color in which she describes an Archaic Triad based primarily on Light (white or light clay ground), Dark (blue, black), and Red (which can be light or dark).[124] Numerous studies of Greek literature and philosophy have shown that dark/light is an important polarity underlying Greek thought. In addition to describing hue, many Greek color terms can also be used to express this contrast. For example, the term κελαινος, used to describe wind, blood, freshly plowed earth, and water, best translates as *dark*.[125] The ancient Greek emphasis on light and dark in poetry rather than on hues as the organizing principle of color, indicated by words for specific colors such as red, blue, etc., even led earlier generations of scholars to propose that the Greeks were color-blind.[126] Such scholars were frustrated by the Greeks' habit of identifying many objects—which in modern Western color vocabularies are given distinct color terms—under one color name. Yet these are literary constructs, just as vases are artistic constructs of an ideological reality. A fourth-century inventory of actual fabric dedicated at Brauron lists a variety of colors rather than emphasizing the light/dark polarity that is so emphasized in literature and art.[127]

---

122. V. Manzelli, "La Policromia Nella Statuaria Greca Arcaica," especially 285. Contra see V. Brinkmann, "Die Farben der Archaischen und Frühklassischen Skulptur," in V. Brinkmann, *Bunte Götter, Die Farbigkeit Antike Skulptur*, 46 and Note 89.

123. J. Gage, *Color and Meaning, Art, Science, and Symbolism* (Berkeley: University of California Press, 1999), 34.

124. E. Walter-Karydi, "Prinzipien der archaischen Farbgebung," in *Studien Zur Klassischen Archäologie, Festschrift für Friedrich Hiller*, ed. F. Hiller and K. Braun (Saarbrücken, 1986), 28.

125. M. Platnauer, "Greek Colour-Perception," *Classical Quarterly*, Vol. 15, No. 3/4 (July–Oct. 1921): 153–54. See also J. Lyons, "The Vocabulary of Color with Particular Reference to Ancient Greek and Classical Latin," in T. Loden, *The Language of Color in the Mediterranean* (Stockholm: Almquist & Wiksell International, 1999), 58.

126. E. Irwin, *Colour Terms in Greek Poetry*, 11.

127. L. Cleland, "The Semiosis of Description: Some Research on Fabric and Colour in the Brauron Inven-

These observations explain why male/female color differentiation would be acceptable in Greece. But to return to our original question: Are there factors specific to Athenian society that cause this distinction to be so consistently observed in Attic black figure? The Athenian insistence that the men of their city were autochthonous—they were sprung directly from the earth—provides an added message of difference between men and women. The mythological first kings of the city—Cecrops, Erectheus, and Erichtonios—are all said to have sprung from the earth, neatly abnegating any reproductive role for women. They are creatures completely different from this subsequently manufactured product, woman. While the goddess of their city is nominally female, she is in many ways more closely identified with the male. She was born not from her mother's womb but from her father's head, and as a virgin she eschews the reproductive function of women.

We can also see specific legislation restricting the activities of women in the city. According to Plutarch (21.5 and 21.4), Solon initiated legislation that curtailed one of women's previously most important roles. They were allowed to give the funerary lament but were limited to the house and the graveside, and women under sixty could not take part in the most public part of the funeral, the funeral procession, unless the relative was a second cousin or closer. Women had to walk behind the men. In addition, an office was established to enforce women's proper public behavior, including activities at festivals.[128] The true seclusion was not from the outdoors, but from participation in the public political life of the city. Legally women had no role in government and no part in the growth of a democratic form of government whose roots lie in the "middling" ideology, in which the most privileged member was the male citizen. In addition, with the Peisistratid revision of Homer taking place during this period, the white-armed women he describes would have been part of Athenian consciousness.

A challenge to the idea that male/female color differentiation on Attic black-figure vases reflects Athenian attitudes toward women comes from our lack of understanding of the audience for these vases. We have seen that in the

tories," in *The Clothed Body in the Ancient World*, ed. L. Cleland, M. Harlow, and L. Llewellyn-Jones (Oxford: Oxbow Books, 2005), 87–95. The list includes a variety of colors including saffron and quince.

128. On this point see M. D. Stansbury-O'Donnell, *Vase Painting, Gender and Social Identity in Archaic Athens*, 219, and S. Pomeroy, *Goddesses, Whores, Wives and Slaves*, 57, who suggests that "women are a perennial source of friction among men. Solon's solution to this problem was to keep them out of sight and to limit their influence."

Geometric period there is a clear connection between aristocratic tastes, expressed through wealthy burials, and the imagery on the vases. Scholars have generally linked many of the Attic black-figure vases to the aristocratic world of the symposium. Kraters, cups, and so on are usually considered the equipment necessary for the all-male drinking party.[129] Would or could vase painters have presented images that spoke to other categories of society? This point has come under particular scrutiny in the work of Sian Lewis, who, based on the fact that the find-spot of a majority of Attic vases is Etruria, considers black figure to be a product designed primarily for the Etruscan export market.[130] The images we so closely scrutinize to uncover Athenian social patterns would thus be more reflective of Etruscan mores and demands than of an Athenian audience. In particular, Lewis points to the fact that despite much scrutiny scholars have been unable to determine the status of women depicted on Attic vases. Especially there seem to be no hard-and-fast iconographic criteria that we can detect for determining who is a respectable Athenian woman and who fits into the class of prostitute or hetaira.

While we are dealing with a different world than that of the monumental tomb art of Egypt, which was clearly commissioned by and for elites, I do not think we can totally divorce Attic black-figure vase-painting imagery from Athens. Male/female color differentiation is particularly apropos to this discussion since it occurs across the board on Attic vases, both on those found at home and on those exported to Etruria. This suggests that we may be asking the wrong question when we wonder whether any given female figure is respectable. The important distinction for the Athenians was not between categories of woman, but between the very category "woman" and the category "male." Male/female color differentiation makes this distinction vividly clear. All females are different from all males and belong to a separate category of being.

Of course not only men used vases. Athenian women gathered water in hydriae and used all manner of other vessels. Would an Athenian woman have had a positive feeling about the differences between male and female emphasized on these vases? Would she have seen in them a model for her own correct behavior, or would she have chafed at underlying misogyny? Literary evidence

---

129. On this connection see, for example, R. T. Neer, *Style and Politics in Athenian Vase-Painting: The Craft of Democracy, ca. 530–460 B.C.E.* (Cambridge: Cambridge University Press, 2002), 10.

130. S. Lewis, *The Athenian Woman.* Contra see C. Reusser, *Vasen für Etrurien: Verbreitung und Funktionen attischer Keramik im Etrurien des 6. Und 5. Jahrhunderts vor Christus* (Zurich: Akanthus, 2002).

is both produced by and addresses primarily an audience of elite males, and even if other members of society are mentioned their lives are still being presented through the eyes of that group. They would seem to control the imagery although not in any formally organized way. While we cannot pinpoint a specific mechanism in place, I agree with Robert Sutton when he states:

> Although it is unclear to what extent the social attitudes depicted on Attic pottery reflect the personal views of individual vase-painters rather than the taste of purchasers, either Athenian or foreign, surely vase-painters planning to market their wares could not have strayed far from what their public (or publics) would tolerate.[131]

The ubiquity of male/female color differentiation in Attic black figure suggests that this construct was widely accepted in Athenian society. Attic black-figure vases consistently mark women as different regardless of the setting or whether the women are mortal or divine. White (i.e., pale) skin provides the clearest signal. The message is that women are fundamentally different from men, not only in their respective spheres of activity but also in their very nature, an alien race living in the midst of men. We have seen in Egypt (Chapter 2) that when the underlying ideology changes, so too does the use of color as gender indicator. The art of the reigns of Hatshepsut and Akhenaten demonstrates this clearly. When, as in the case of Hatshepsut, the role of pharaoh is occupied by a woman, dark skin is used for the female ruler rather than the light skin traditional for women. When, under Akhenaten, a new religious view is imposed, male and female are both painted dark. If, as the evidence of literature, archaeology, and political discourse presented in this chapter shows, Greek use of male/female color differentiation is linked to underlying ideas about women, why do the Greeks abandon this convention with the invention of red figure? Do ideas about women change, or is something else at work? The next chapter explores these questions. The operative word here is *explores*. Definitive answers are difficult.

131. R. F. Sutton, "The Good, the Base and the Ugly: The Drunken Orgy in Attic Vase Painting and the Athenian Self," in B. Cohen, ed., *Not the Classical Ideal*, 181.

CHAPTER 4

Greece

The Exception that Proves the Rule— Attic Red Figure

While black figure with its added white for female flesh continues to be produced throughout the history of Athenian vase painting, it loses its status as the dominant Athenian vase painting form to a new technique which first appears around 530 BC. Developed in the Athenian potter's quarter, red figure reverses the standard schema of black figures against a reserved clay background. Now, rather than shiny black silhouettes against a red clay background, figures are the red clay, reserved against a shiny black background. Details are no longer incised, as in black figure, but are instead "drawn" with a relief line composed of dilute clay as seen in Figures 22 and 23. No radical new technical developments are needed to create red figure; the shiny black color and the reserved orange clay are the products of firing. Most important for our study is the abandonment of added white for women's flesh. Unlike black figure, both men and women are now the same color—the orange of the fired clay.

Is the new one-color system representative of deeper issues involving the status of women in the late Archaic period? Are other factors at work? Are aesthetics or even technical considerations, rather than symbolism, driving this change? What forces were at work in the last quarter of the sixth century BC that made it acceptable to depict men and women without differentiating them by skin color?

These are complex questions and we are limited by a lack of literary sources that deal specifically with the late Archaic period (530–490 BC). For the subsequent Classical period (5th century–4th c. BC), when red figure is the dominant style of vase painting, our sources make it clear that the ideas concerning the nature of women as different—and dangerous—creatures of the interior

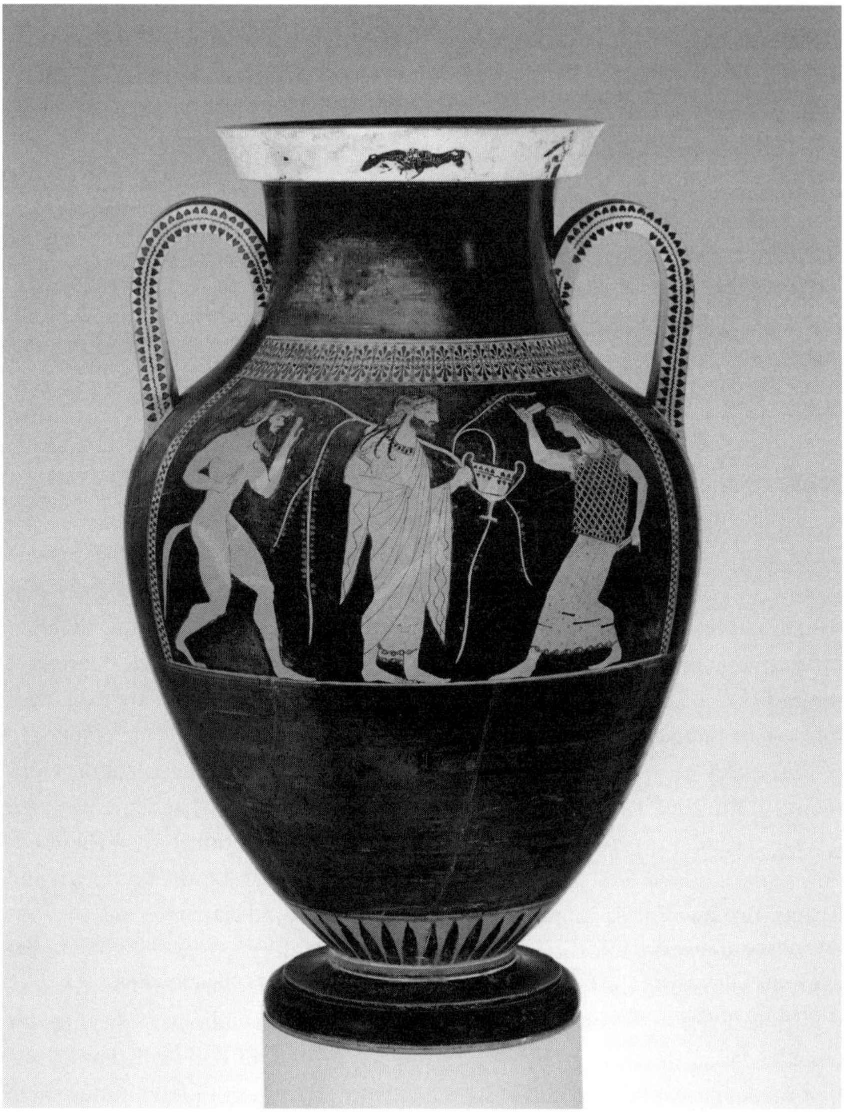

Fig. 22. Terracotta amphora (jar). Andokides Painter (sixth century BC) Reverse: Dionysos between satyr and maenad Greek, Attic, ca. 530 BC. Terracotta, h. 22 5/8 in (57.5 cm). Purchase, Joseph Pulitzer bequest, 1963 (63.11.6). (The Metropolitan Museum of Art, New York, NY, U.S.A. Image © The Metropolitan Museum of Art/Art Resource, NY.)

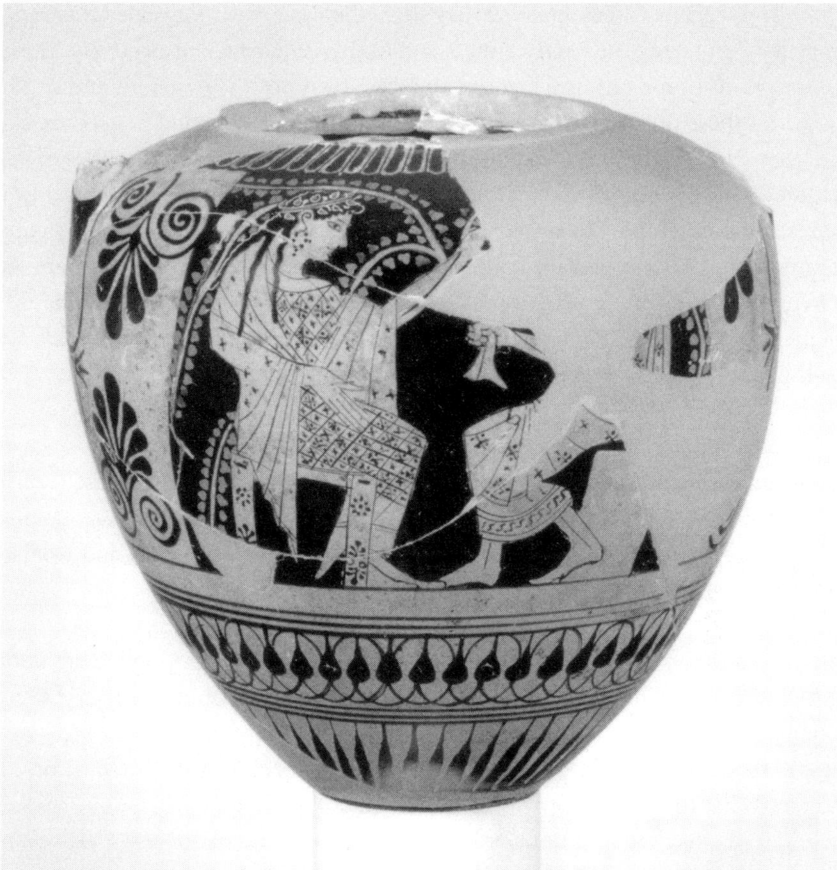

Fig. 23. Two-handled jar (amphora). Three-line group. Greek, Archaic Period, about 525 BC. Place of manufacture: Greece, Attica, Athens. Ceramic red figure. Height: 5 5/16 in (13.5 cm); diameter: 5 1/2 in (14 cm). (Museum of Fine Arts, Boston. Francis Bartlett Donation of 1900, 03.790.)

have not changed. In fact the rhetoric of seclusion is, if anything, even stronger than in earlier periods.

Indeed, most of the literary sources which have been used by modern scholars to support the actuality of female seclusion date to this period. In particular, household interiors are described as separated by gender. In, for example, Xenophon's *Oikonomikos* 9.2–5 and Lysisas I, 9–10, two terms—*andron* and *gunaikon*—occur which, because they share the root words for male (*aner*) and female (*gyne*), are translated as men's and women's quarters, respectively. These descriptions of the physical layout of houses stress both segregation and seclusion. Yet these divisions prove very difficult to find when actual houses are excavated. The lack of preserved houses from Athens hinders the discussion, but studies of Greek houses have shown that there are consistent architectural features across regions.[1] Excavated classical houses, which would be roughly contemporary with the literary sources, reveal no separate area for women. At Olynthus, for example, the domestic spatial pattern seems instead to be designed to restrict access to outsiders rather than to divide male from female within the house. As Nevett argues (pp. 173–79):

> Athens is likely to have been similar to Greek cities elsewhere. . . . the principal form of house considered here, the single-entrance courtyard house, was a product of social pressures which required the separation of female family members from male guests, rather than a division between men and women per se.[2]

The only gender-specific separate area that can be identified is a room which excavators identify as a male dining room. While objects which can be connected with female activity—toiletries, weaving implements, etc.—are found throughout the house, one area is set aside specifically for men.[3] Corner suggests that the andron provides a sanctioned imposition of the public (male) world into what has traditionally been the private (female) domain.[4] This public/private dichotomy, between the domestic world of the female and the legal democratic system of the male and the tensions it creates, is also an important topos in Athenian drama of the Classical period. As Saxonhouse notes: "The city will always be limited by that which it cannot fully assimilate into itself—for the Greeks, in particular, this was the female, sexuality and the family."[5] Plays such as *Antigone* and *Medea* explore this dynamic.

1. L. Nevett, *House and Society in the Ancient Greek World* (Cambridge: Cambridge University Press, 1999), 17–18.
2. Ibid. 173–79.
3. Ibid. 170.
4. S. Corner, "Bringing the Outside In: Civic Sexuality," in A.Glazebrook and M.M. Henry, *Greek Prostitutes in the Ancient Mediterranean, 800 BCE–200 CE* (Madison: The University of Wisconsin Press, 2011), 60–85.
5. A. Saxonhouse, *Fear of Diversity: The Birth of Political Science in Ancient Greek Thought* (Chicago: University of Chicago Press, 1992), x.

In his famous *Funeral Oration*, Perikles pronounces that a woman's character is finest when she "is least talked of among men, whether for good or bad."[6] Thus the rhetoric of the Classical period consistently privileges the world outside the house, since this is where the activities of the fully formed democracy and the lives of the male writers of our ancient sources were conducted. Thus as Robertson states: "Among upper-class fifth-century Athenians the rule that men (athletes, fighters, social beings) belong in the sun, women in the shuttered house, was probably more absolute than at any other time or place in antiquity."[7] Women were not active participants in the democratic government; they could not even vote.

Medical texts also describe fundamental *physiological* differences between men and women. As Dean-Jones showed, menstruation is used as the basis for classifying women's skin as being more porous than men's, which causes them to be, depending upon the ancient source, either hotter or colder than men.[8]

Perhaps the most striking Classical image of women's roles is the chryselephantine statue of Athena housed in the Parthenon. The city's goddess stands on a pedestal depicting the creation of that scourge of mankind, Pandora. Placing the creation of Pandora on the statue base on which the colossal gold and ivory statue of Athena stands emphasizes Athena's differences from the 'race of women.' Pandora is literally beneath the feet of the city's patron goddess, who is not herself necessarily a champion of women. While Athena did give to women the art of weaving, (which can be seen as a double-edged skill allowing women such as Deianira to create deadly cloaks), her birth relied on the co-opting of the traditional female role of child bearer by her father Zeus. She aids young male heroes, such as Herakles and Perseus, and in the oft-quoted passage from the *Oresteia* states that she identifies with the male. As Hurwitt notes, Pandora's presence on the base of Athena's statue serves as a further reminder of the dangerous creatures which live within the city, the women of Athens, who are not sprung from the earth as are the males of the city but are a separate and distinct creation.[9] As Saxonhouse states: "Unifying, ordering, autochthony also demands exclusion of the human female from the origins of

6. Thucydides 2.45, quoted in R. Just, *Women in Athenian Law and Life* (London: Routledge, 1994), 9.
7. M. Robertson, *The Art of Vase-Painting in Classical Athens* (Cambridge: Cambridge University Press, 1992), 8.
8. L. Dean-Jones, *Women's Bodies in Classical Greek Science* (Oxford: Oxford University Press, 1994), 55–6; temperature: 44.
9. J. Hurwitt, "Beautiful Evil: Pandora and the Athena Parthenos," *American Journal of Archaeology*, 99:2, 171–86.

the city. The city and its public space is the realm of male rulers who have sprung from the earth."[10]

Indeed, Xenophon's *Oecnomicus* suggests that during this period the ideal can even become real. Ischomachos describes his wife's use of make-up to add to her allure. "She had applied a great deal of white lead to her face, that she might seem fairer than she was."[11] In the Greek theater the male actors who portrayed female characters wore white masks to mark their identify as women. Male/female color differentiation would fit in perfectly as the visual manifestation of the ideas outlined above, and yet red figure abandons it. We need to return to the beginnings of red figure to examine what circumstances may have contributed to this significant departure from previous iconography.

First, as we noted, red figure is one of a number of experiments with vase decoration developed in the Athenian potter's quarter around 530 BC. Its invention is often attributed to the Andokides painter.[12] This painter's interest in experimentation can be seen on a vase depicting women (Amazons?) arming on one side and nude women shown swimming on the other.[13] The vase is produced in a unique technique in which the black background of red figure is combined with a layer of white ground so that the reserve figures are not the red color of fired clay typical of red figure but are, instead, white. This is not a question of added white, but rather 'reserve' white.[14] As mentioned above, the figures depicted are all women. This appears to be a one-of-a-kind vase, so perhaps it cannot be relied upon too much, but the fact that all of the figures are women and that an unusual technique was tried to provide them all with the traditional white skin suggests that even the inventor of red figure was still interested in white for female flesh. It might be equally plausible that the Andokides Painter created this special vase because he found that added white paint did not adhere to reserved clay of red figure in the same way that it did in black figure and was searching for a solution. However, the fact that, as we shall see, later (fifth-century) Attic and South Italian vases make copious use of

10. A. W. Saxonhouse, *Fear of Diversity*, 52. See also H.A. Shapiro, "Autochthony and the Visual Arts," in D.Boedecker and K.A. Raaflaub, *Democracy and the Arts in Fifth-Century Athens* (Cambridge: Harvard University Press, 1998), 127–51.

11. Xenophon, *Oeconomicus*, x.2, quoted in J. Jenkins and V. Turner, *The Greek Body* (Los Angeles: J.Paul Getty Museum, 2009), 20.

12. J. G. Pedley, *Greek Art and Archaeology* (London: Prentice Hall, 1998), 195.

13. White-figured Amphora of Type A, Paris, Musée du Louvre F 203, J. D. Beazley, *Attic Black-Figure Vase-Painters* (Oxford 1956), 253.middle.3 , B. Cohen, ed., *The Colors of Clay*, Catalogue Number 51, with illustration.

14. J. R. Mertens, "White Ground," in B. Cohen, ed., *The Colors of Clay*, 197–98.

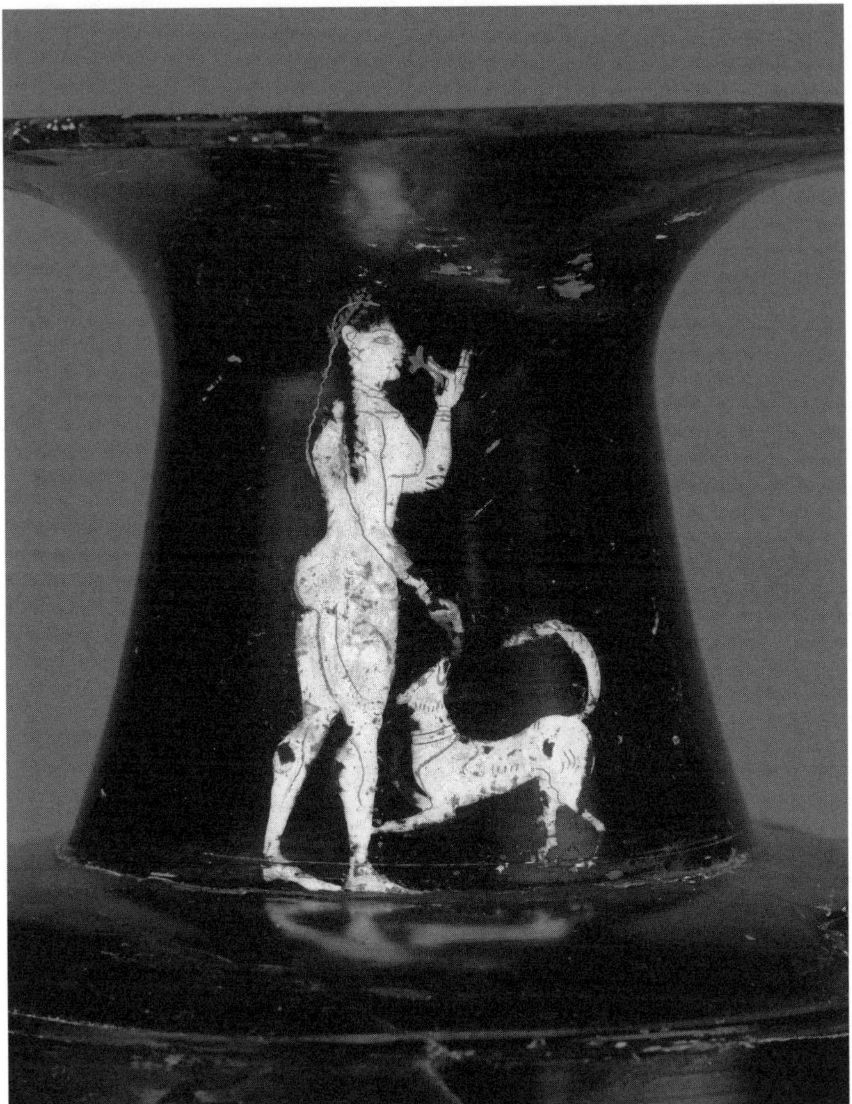

Fig. 24. Detail from a black and white neck-amphora. Nikosthenes Painter (sixth century BC) and Painter N (late sixth century BC). Woman smelling a flower and caressing a dog. h. 32 cm. F114. (Photo: Hervé Lewandowski. Louvre, Paris, France. Photo Credit: Réunion des Musées Nationaux/Art Resource, NY.)

added white suggests that this was probably not a major problem. We did see (in Chapter 3) that an earlier painter, the Amasis painter, employed outline for some of his female figures. At first glance the fact that they (female figures) are left the reserve color of the clay does resemble later red figure. However, color contrast is maintained because the male figures are the shiny black glaze of black figure.

Among the other techniques developed at the same time as red figure are coral red (shiny red-gloss background), Six's technique (red or white silhouette figures are painted over the fired shiny black vase) as in Figure 24, and white ground (the entire surface of the vase is covered with white slip and the figures are drawn in outline or a variation in which black-figure silhouettes decorate white ground).[15] Other than red figure and white ground, these are short-lived techniques with varying uses of male/female color differentiation. For example, in Six's technique figural decoration is created by painting over a black glaze background. Male figures are painted the orange color, which in red figure is created through reserving areas during the firing process. Alternatively, in this technique the outline of male figures can be incised. The result is a black silhouette outlined in the red color of the fired clay against a shiny black background, resulting in a figure with black skin.[16] Women, on the other hand, are painted white over the shiny black glaze. So, for example, a nude woman (painted white) is depilated by a satyr (black glaze and outline) on a lekythos in Basel.[17] Males can also be painted with added white. We can see this on a skyphos in Malibu which depicts a young man drinking (from a skyphos),[18] but in these cases all of the figural decoration is in added white, suggesting that this is more of an attempt at emulating the light-on-dark scheme of red figure, rather than following the principles of male/female gender differentiation. Thus we see a great deal of variety in vase painting during this period and exploration of new types of decoration has to be counted among the factors that influenced the change to red figure.

All of the new methods of decoration which we discussed above have suggested to some scholars that vase painters may have felt restricted by black fig-

---

15. Ibid. for copious illustrations.
16. See, for example, a lekythos, New York Metropolitan Museum of Art 67, 11.22, Rogers Fund 1967. B. Cohen, "Six's Technique: Black Ground," in B. Cohen, ed., *The Colors of Clay*, No. 23, 98–99.
17. Basel Antikenmuseum Basel und Sammlung Ludwig BS 423. B. Cohen "Six's Technique: Black Ground," in B. Cohen, ed., *The Colors of Clay*, No. 25, 102–3.
18. J. Paul Getty Museum 76 AE 127 in B. Cohen, "Six's Technique: Black Ground," B. Cohen, ed., *The Colors of Clay*, No. 21, 94–95.

ure and wanted to try something new, that in fact they felt the need to break free from the constraints imposed by the black-figure silhouette technique in which details were rendered by incision. Since red figure appears at the same time that sculptors are beginning to explore new ways of depicting the human body, with greater emphasis on accurate depiction of musculature and anatomy as well as more challenging poses than previously attempted, some scholars stress the connection to these new ideas.[19] Thus, according to this theory red figure was invented to exploit a new interest in naturalism.

However, Neer has shown that while many of these new spatial possibilities are inherent in red figure, they are not exploited in the earliest red-figure vases which exhibit no more ambitious poses or understanding of musculature than their black-figure predecessors.[20] Instead, rather than initially being interested in anatomical realism, red figure in its early phase remains very much a technique still invested in silhouette. Again, what has changed is the background against which the silhouette appears. As Cohen notes, the effect of red figure is still very much a silhouette, not an outline technique.[21] The silhouette is the reserve color of the clay rather than the black, but the shiny black that now becomes the background limits any attempt at drawing beyond the contours of the figure's silhouette. Interest in the relationship between figures and the background is also shown in the type of sculpture which is usually considered most closely related stylistically to vase painting, namely relief sculpture. Around 530 BC the color of the sculptural background is changed from red to blue.[22] This is not the reversal of dark on light that we see in vase painting, but it is a shift to a color that could be seen as more natural. Rather than the impenetrable background suggested by the previous use of red for relief sculpture, we now have a greater sense of all-encompassing space provided by the suggestion of the sky inherent in blue. Yet while here the shift in background color implies limitless space, the same cannot truly be said of red figure. As Boardman notes, ". . . the

---

19. For example, M. Robertson, *The Art of Vase-painting in Classical Athens* (Cambridge: Cambridge University Press, 2002), 32–34.
20. R. Neer, *Style and Politics in Athenian Vase-Painting* (Cambridge: Cambridge University Press, 2002), 32–34.
21. B. Cohen, "Outline as a Special Technique in Black and Red-figure Vase-Painting," in B. Cohen, ed., *The Colors of Clay*, 151.
22. On this change see E. Walter-Karydi, "Prinzipien der archaischen Farbgebung," in *Studien zur klassischen Archaölogie* (Festschrift für Friedrich Hiller), ed. K . Braun and A. Furtwangler (Saarbrucken 1986), 29. B.S. Ridgway, Prayers in Stone, *Greek Architectural Sculpture* (Chicago: Ares Publishing, 1993), 110; on the comparison between red figure and relief, see J. Boardman, *Athenian Red Figure Vases: The Archaic* Period (London: Thames and Hudson, 1985), 14.

effect of the black ground which removed all possibility of rendering depth of field [which in this craft] meant that even the simplest perspective was not attempted. The figures stand spot-lighted on a narrow stage."[23] Experiments in the relationship of figure to background are very much in the air during this period, although the change in the contrast between the two elements results in different effects in sculpture and red figure.

Although Andokides is credited with the invention of red figure, the next generation of red-figure vase painters (510–490 BC) fully exploits the possibilities of complex poses in space inherent in the new technique. Unlike the initial red-figure artists, these vase painters, labeled by scholars "the Pioneers," attempt complex three-quarter and twisting poses and even brag about their skill in asides to each other written on their vases. On one vase by Euthymides, for example, he boasts "as never Euphronios," suggesting that his skill exceeds that of his fellow vase painter.[24] No longer do we see the frontal torsos with profile legs and heads characteristic of the stiff silhouettes of black figure. As Cohen notes, "In general, the red-figure painter enthusiastically seeks to reflect the details and dynamics of life, while the black-figure painter creates rigid, hieratic forms that are traditional rather than convincing."[25] This dynamic quality is perhaps aided by the use of the relief line in red figure, which is a drawing rather than an incising technique and is thus closer to the style of wall painting. Preserved wall would be invaluable in showing if male/female color differentiation persists in that medium during this period, but we have nothing from Athens. We do have a painted tomb from Paestum—the "Tomb of the Diver."[26] Male figures are shown banqueting. They are painted tan rather than reddish brown. In addition, a male diver painted inside the tomb is the typical dark reddish brown. However, without women in the scene it is difficult to see whether a strong contrast was employed. A less sharp color distinction between male and female appears on one of the few preserved examples of painting on a much earlier Archaic panel painting from Pitsa, showing women and a boy making offerings at an altar. The women's flesh is left the white slip color of the panel and the boy is painted a slightly darker tan.[27] Of course, the color palette is also more expansive than red figure, with clothing painted in blue, red, and

23. J. Boardman, *Athenian Red Figure Vases: The Archaic Period*, 14.
24. Attic red-figure amphora by Euthymides. Stattliche Antikensamlungen. J. Boardman, *Athenian Red Figure Vases*, 29
25. B. Cohen, "Bilingual Vases and Vase-Painters," in B. Cohen, ed., *The Colors of Clay*, 30.
26. Paestum Museum, J. G. Pedley, *Greek Art and Archaeology*, 247, Figs. 7.48 and 7.49.
27. Pitsa plaques: E. Walter-Karydi, "Prinzipien der archaisshcen Farbegung," 25, pl. 2 and 3.

green. These paintings are generally identified as representatives of Corinthian painting, so we cannot necessarily say that Attic paintings of the same period would use such a muted contrast.

Returning to red figure, it is clear that the work of the Pioneers personifies the interest in more naturalistic poses and facial features characteristic of the sculpture of the Late Archaic period. The so-called "archaic smile," which was the standard facial expression regardless of the situation in which the figure was placed, is gone. Eye shape is no longer used to distinguish between men and women. Indeed the profile eye is no longer as common. Instead the pupil is moved forward from the center of the eye and the corner is open.[28] Thus male/female color differentiation could be counted among the unrealistic features that are abandoned during this period.

In the preceding chapter I argued that rather than being a realistic reflection of relative sun exposure male/female color differentiation is, in fact, an artistic device that reflects underlying beliefs about the role and statue of women. If male/female color differentiation reflects reality, we are left with the paradox that when vase-painting images are considered to be most naturalistic, an artistic feature, which as you will recall is traditionally described in the scholarship as natural, is not retained. Indeed Robertson suggests that red figure "allowed developments in drawing the human face and form to be carried on in figures of both sexes."[29] We can thus see that contrary to previous scholars' ideas that male/female color differentiation reflects a "natural" sun exposure it is, in fact, the abandonment of this convention that shows figures at their most natural.

However, the trajectory of red-figure style cautions us to remember that this naturalism was not necessarily intentional. In its earliest phase, as we have noted, red figure is very much a silhouette-driven experiment rather than an attempt at naturalism. However, its persistence and ever-increasing popularity as the métier for the best vase painters suggests that its retention is congruent with some societal ideas. In addition, the rise of another medium, bronze, may have made the common color scheme for male and female flesh seem appropriate as well. While large-scale bronze sculpture is primarily a phenomenon of the Classical period, the late Archaic period saw an increase in the number of small bronze statues, many of which were dedicated and in full view on the

28. J. Boardman, *Athenian Red Figure Vases*, 17.
29. M. Robertson, *The Art of Vase-Painting in Classical Athens*, 8.

Athenian Acropolis.[30] Unlike their larger counterparts, which tended to emulate stiffer early forms such as Kouroi, these statuettes exhibited a variety of poses similar to the exploitation of the body in motion found on the vases of the Pioneers.[31] More importantly, the bronzes provide a similar commonality of skin color. Bronze statues, whether they depict men or women, carry a uniform patina; thus, as in red figure, male and female have the same skin color. Since marble continues to be the preferred medium for larger-scale sculpture—votive, architectural, and funerary—it would be informative to know if the color convention is abandoned in stone sculpture as it was in red figure. Brinkman's examination of the architectural relief sculpture of the Siphnian Treasury frieze uncovered traces of reddish brown on the flesh of several of the male figures.[32] Lack of color on the females could indicate that they were left the white color of the marble. Brinkmann reconstructs the later Archer of the c. 490-BC west pediment of the temple of Aphaia from Aegina as having a very light pinkish tan color.[33]

An unusual vase-painting example may indicate that male flesh could continue to be painted reddish brown for free-standing stone sculpture. A rhyton (statuette) vase in the British Museum dated to c. 500–490 BC is composed of a seated bearded male figure (usually identified as Dionysos) modeled from clay as a statuette holding a red-figure drinking horn.[34] Figures on the drinking horn are painted in the typical red-figure style with no male/female color differentiation. However, the Dionysos statuette is covered with an added layer of red paint. Thus, while the drinking horn follows typical red-figure style, the added paint for the sculpted Dionysus might suggest that his sculptural form required a color scheme associated with stone sculpture. This is a frail vessel to support a strong case for the coloration of sculpture, but if it does represent marble coloration we would have red figure and bronze sculpture on the cutting edge, while traditional black figure and marble sculpture would be following a more conservative approach by continuing to mark gender through color.

30. C. M. Keesling, *The Votive Statues of the Athenian Acropolis* (Cambridge: Cambridge University Press, 2003), 71–93.
31. On this point see C. Mattusch, *Greek Bronze Statuary from the Beginnings through the Fifth c. B.C.* (Ithaca: Cornell University Press, 1988), 86 and 99.
32. V. Brinkmann, *Beobachtungen zum formalin Aufbau und zum Zinngehalt der Friese des Siphnierschautzhauses* (Munich: Ennepetal, 1994), 49.
33. V. Brinkmann, *Di Polychromie der Archaischen und Früklassischen Skulptur* (Munich: Biering and Brinkmann, 20030 43, No. 281).
34. London, The British Museum GR 1873. 8–20. M. True, "Athenian Potters and the Production of Plastic Vases," in B. Cohen, *The Colors of Clay*, Cat. No. 77, 264–65.

White ground, the other long-lived new technique developed during the late Archaic period, presents a slightly different picture. Its name refers to the background color of the vase, but, as noted above, the figures themselves can be depicted by the black-figure technique or by outline drawing.[35] When the figures are black figure, male/female color differentiation is not used. This is also initially the case for those decorated with outline drawing as well; men and women are drawn in outline and their flesh is left as the white background color. However, although the term "white" suggests that the background is the same tone as that used in black figure to denote female flesh, the actual color is closer to cream than to bright white. Around 490 BC there is a short-lived series of vases in which an additional application of white paint is used on female figures even though the use of outline against the white slip of the background already makes their flesh white. The added "second white" is in fact a truer white. We shall return to this development later, but for now will continue our examination of the changes in the last quarter of the sixth century.

As noted above, of the many experimental techniques developed in the Athenian potter's quarter in the Late Archaic period, the two with the greatest longevity and volume of production are red figure and white ground (with red figure produced in by far the greatest quantity). Both of these techniques abandon dark/light male/female color differentiation. Why should techniques whose color formula contradicts what was the most basic iconographical distinction in vase painting (male vs. female) become the dominant forms? We have already seen that artistic and technical experimentation certainly led to the creation of these styles and that a common color for male and female fits with the growing interest in more lifelike forms found in sculpture during this period. Thus a partial answer to the question posed earlier in this chapter is that an increased interest in naturalistic depictions would seem to support the abandonment of male/female color differentiation in red-figure vase painting. Yet in earlier chapters of this book I argued for clear links between the use of the convention in the first place and societal attitudes about women. The sharp black/white color contrast visually marks the Ancient Athenian view of women and men as opposite polarities. White represented an ideological seclusion of

---

35. On White Ground see J. R. Mertens, *Attic White-Ground. Its Development on Shapes other than Lekythoi* (New York: Garland, 1977); I. Weihgartner, *Attische Weisgrunde Keramik. Maltechniken, Werkstätten, Formen, Verwendung* (Mainz: Von Zabern, 1983); U. Koch-Brinkmann, *Polychrome Bilder auf Weisgrundigen Lekythen* (Munich: Biering and Brinkmann, 1999); J. H. Oakley, *Picturing Death in Classical Athens: the Evidence of the White Lekythoi* (New York: Cambridge University Press, 2004).

women, a connection between females and the domestic (interior) world rather than the political (exterior) world. Does the lack of color differentiation between males and females in red figure represent a change in those views?

When looking at what we know of this period, no evidence supports the idea that equality of skin color is equivalent to any other kind of social equality. There is general scholarly agreement that there is no historical support for the idea that the end of the Archaic period marks a time of equality for women.[36] On the contrary, Straus states, "Athenians arguably created a culture that made even poor citizen males feel part of a privileged elite: poor they might be, but because they were masters of their women, no man, not even a rich man, could threaten their dignity and honor."[37] Yet this does not mean that there are not tensions surrounding issues of gender which might be consonant with red figure's growing popularity and its abandonment of color as gender indicator.

The Late Archaic period is a time of great change in Athens as the city moves from the tyranny of the Peisistratids to the fully established democracy of the Classical period. In addition, new external threats arise, in particular the increasing involvement of the Persian empire in Greece. As others have noted, this is a time of intense scrutiny of what it means to be an Athenian citizen-male.[38] Kleisthenes' reforms of c.509/8 BC extended citizenship to a broader segment of the male citizen body than had previously held it. Status within society which had been dependent on aristocratic pedigree and/or wealth was changing to one in which, theoretically at least, all citizen males were equal. As Stewart states:

> At a stroke, then, Kleistehenes simultaneously created a public sphere in Athenian politics that was predicated upon a particular notion of social justice (*dike*), was independent of place and person, and was dominated by the city at its center. The polis was now a signifying space where a theoretical equality of

36. There is a lengthy bibliography on Athenian women. A good in-depth survey is R. Just, *Women in Athenian Law and Life* (London: Routledge, 1989); for a suggestion that things might not have been as bad as traditionally portrayed by scholars, see B. S. Strauss, "Ideology and Society in Democratic Athens," in *Archaeological Institute of America Colloquia and Conference Papers. No. 2: Democracy 2500? Questions and Challenges*, eds. I. Morris and K. A. Raaflaub (Dubuque: Kendall/Hunt Publishing, 1997).
37. B. S. Strauss, "Ideology and Society in Democratic Athens," 147.
38. R. F. Sutton, "The Good , the Base and the Ugly: the Drunken Orgy in Attic Vase Painting and the Athenian Self," in *Not the Classical Ideal: Athens and the Construction of the Other in Greek Art*, ed. B. Cohen (Leiden: Brill Academic Publishers, 2000), 180–202. R. T. Neer, *Greek Art and Archaeology, A New History c. 2500–150 BCE* (New York: Thames and Hudson, 2012), 208–9.

> rights or *isonomia* prevailed that transcended the individual and his parochial concerns.[39]

In addition, increasing use of the phalanx formed in tribal cohorts added to the egalitarianism of military activity.[40] This combination of newly enfranchised members of society and the ideology of *isonomia* altered the previous standards for the evaluation of male status.

During this critical period, not only are the decorative techniques of vase painting the subject of experimentation, but also the subject matter. Several new and short-lived themes appear to provide a method of working out some of the new societal tensions. In the work of the Pioneers, the group of red-figure vase-painters whose floruit corresponds to Kleisthenes and the burgeoning democracy, Neer notes that not only is self-referential rivalry apparent, as we saw in the "as never Euthymides" message on the vase by Euphronios, but there is also social commentary. Some Pioneer Group vases depict occasions such as the symposium, the traditional preserve of aristocrats, in which some of the participants are labeled with the names of the vase painters or potters themselves.[41] This would be a deliberate tweaking of the old status rules, in which the symposium was the prerogative of the aristocratic male. Another indicator of the working out of status during this time is the appearance in red figure of images of ugly and deformed individuals in graphic orgy scenes. Sutton infers that ". . . this spirit can be understood as a weapon in a kind of cultural war in Athens during the sixth century: Recently empowered social groups that had been marginalized in the old order, including craftsmen and traders, challenged established aristocratic values as the polis moved toward the egalitarian ideals of the Classical democracy."[42]

The Acropolis votive statues provide an intriguing corollary to the vase-painting evidence. In that group of monuments there is a distinct increase in dedications in the period from 510–480 BC. Uniquely among sanctuary dedications, those from the Acropolis sometimes list the occupation of the dedicator as a craftsman or manual laborer. This combination of increased volume of dedication and the presumed lower class status of some dedicators has led to

39. A. Stewart, *Art, Desire and the Body in Ancient Greece* (Cambridge: Cambridge University Press, 1997), 138.
40. A. Snodgrass, *Archaic Greece: the Age of Experiment* (London: J.M. Dent and Sons, Ltd., 1980), 151.
41. R. T. Neer, *Style and Politics in Athenian Vase Painting*, 133–34 (list).
42. R. F. Sutton, "The Good, the Base and the Ugly," in B. Cohen, ed., *Not the Classical Ideal: Athens and the Construction of the Other in Greek Art*, 200.

the assumption that Kleisthenes' reforms of 509/8 allowed these individuals to usurp what had been an aristocratic privilege as has been suggested for the symposium scenes on the red-figure vases of the Pioneers. Keesling, in her thorough reconsideration of these monuments, rejects this connection, pointing out that both the dating of the monuments and the identity of the dedicators are by no means as secure as they are usually taken to be. Also, the number of dedications actually decreases after the establishment of the full-blown democracy, and this is not due to a replacement of private monuments with public ones as is sometimes attested.[43] Are we, perhaps, trying to wring too much out of the evidence in an attempt to connect objects (vases, statues) dated on the bases of relative stylistic chronology to the more 'absolute' chronology of historical events? I think that taken together, despite the holes in the evidence, they do support the idea that something is changing in Athenian society during this period. Connecting this change with Kleisthenes' reforms does not seem to me to be out of the range of possibility. Again with red figure we are talking about a response to societal trends, not to a fiat that implements a new artistic program.

Thus status issues of males *vis a vis* one another may have become the dominant polarity expressed in vase painting rather than the previous male/female dichotomy. In addition to these internal status issues, there is also a growing external threat in the form of increasingly contentious relationship between Athens and the Persian Empire. While the Persian invasion of Athens in 480 is a critical moment, tensions had been developing for some time. Earlier Persian involvement with the cities of Ionia during the Late Archaic period 520–490 BC leading to Athenian support of the Ionian revolt had already placed Athens in a state of apprehension about this foreign threat. Thus an external threat may have become a factor in emphasizing Athenian solidarity. What it means to be an Athenian comes to be defined not only internally but against the rest of the world.

While it is true that the post-invasion Classical period provides the greatest number of vase-painting and other images of 'barbarian' others,[44] a striking example of contrast between Athenians and foreigners is also found on red-figure head vases. A few vase painters begin to use skin color as a distinguishing ethnic feature for one foreign group—Ethiopians. I use the term *Ethiopian* because that is the term the ancient Greeks used. Trying to apply outdated racial

43. C. M. Keesling, *The Votive Statues of the Athenian Acropolis* (Cambridge: Cambridge University Press, 2003), 60–63.
44. On this see M. Miller, "The Myth of Bousiris," in Cohen, *Not the Classical Ideal*, 413–41.

categories such as "Negro" to this group only serves to confuse the issue. The name *Ethiopian* itself translates as "burned, black faces" and is applied by the Greeks to all Africans, other than Egyptians, and is not to be confused with the geographic limits of the modern country of Ethiopia.[45] Several Janiform head vases, molded with an outward looking face on each side, clearly emphasize the experimentation with the new polarity which is beginning during the late Archaic period. One such vase (Figure 25) contrasts a red-figure Greek woman with a black shiny glaze Ethiopian man.[46] The contrast is every bit as striking as the previous black-figure white/black skin color differentiation. It has been suggested that this pairing is one of two marginalized types—woman and Ethiopian; however, Herakles is also paired with an Ethiopian in another head vase.[47] Ethiopians are also paired with Scythians in this type of vase. The Ethiopian Scythian topos, with the pairing representing the extremes of human appearance, is also popular in literature.[48] The Ethiopian is but one of the foreigners who begin to be contrasted with Greeks in art. These new polarities are emphasized over the previous male/female polarity of black figure. Margaret Miller has shown that eventually the foreign "other" telescopes into Greek vs. Persian, with most foreigners being given eastern costume.[49]This is not to say that gender anxiety has disappeared. Stewart sees the increase of Amazons on Greek vases during the late Archaic period as a visual method of working out both sets of fears. As Stewart describes them, Amazons are ". . . all too obviously human, conveniently located beyond the Greek world's eastern borders, formidable fighters, and sexually intriguing to boot . . ."[50] They embody the need to defend against the wild, untamed nature of woman and also against the danger of foreign invasion. The fact that they are always defeated by their male opponents reaffirms the correct ordering of both gender relations and international affairs.

These two parallel threads—male status issues and the foreign threat—add

---

45. F. Snowden, Jr., "Greeks and Ethiopians," in *Greeks and Barbarians: Essays on the Interactions between Greeks and non-Greeks and the Consequences for Eurocentrism*, ed. J. Coleman and C. A. Walz (Bethesda, MD: CDL Press, 1997), 103–4.

46. Paris, Musée du Louvre CA 987.

47. For this interpretation see F. Lissarrague, "Identity and Otherness: The Case of Attic Head Vases and Plastic Vases," *Source* 15 No. 1 (1995); See also M. True, "Plastic Vases and Vases with Plastic Additions," in Cohen, *The Colors of Clay*, Catalogue Nos.70–89, 268–73. Herakles Vase: Malibu, J. Paul Getty Museum 83 AE, 218; Snowden, *Blacks in Antiquity*, Fig. 14; M. True, "Plastic Vases and Vases with Plastic Additions," Catalogue No. 81, 272–73.

48. F. Snowden, Jr. *Blacks in Antiquity* (Cambridge: Belknap Press, 1970),vii.

49. M. C. Miller, "The Myth of Bousiris," in *Not the Classical Ideal: Athens and the Construction of the Other in Greek Art*, ed. B. Cohen, 413–41.

50. A. Stewart, "Imag(in)ing the Other: Amazons and Ethnicity in Fifth-Century Athens," *Poetics Today* (1995), 583.

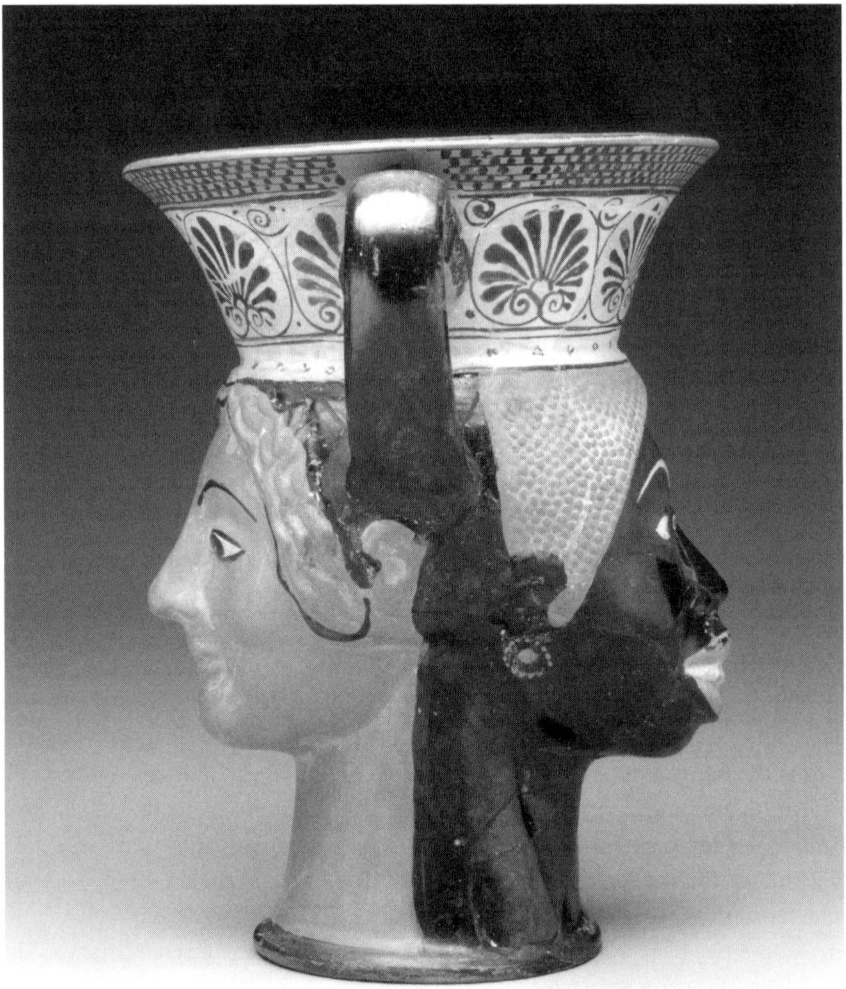

Fig. 25. High-handled drinking cup (kantharos). The London Class. Greek, Late Archaic Period, about 510–480 BC. Place of manufacture: Greece, Attica, Athens. Ceramic, red figure. Height: 7 9/16 in (19.2 cm); diameter: 5 5/8 in (14.3 cm). (Museum of Fine Arts, Boston. Henry Lillie Pierce Fund, 98.926).

to the factors influencing the abandonment of the long-standing convention in vase painting which we discussed above.

This is not to say that red figure was *created* to express these issues, but rather that it became the dominant style because it supported these concepts. Although we can identify broad trends with which the abandonment of male/female color differentiation meshes, determining a specific agent of change is not possible. In Egypt's pharaonically controlled artistic program we saw how color differentiation was manipulated by various rulers to present their particular message. In Greece we are not dealing with a top-down system as in Egypt where a central authority controls the artistic message. It is more a case of particular experiments in vase painting resonating with ideas that are prominent at the time.

In the subsequent Classical period after Athens' important role in the defeat of the Persians (490–480 BC) during the fully established democracy, red figure continues to be the dominant vase-painting style. As we noted in the beginning of this chapter, ideas about female difference and seclusion continue to be emphasized in literature. With the full-fledged democracy, tensions about the place of women continue. As discussed above, the public/private dichotomy between men and women is one of the important themes in tragedy.

Red-figure vase painting does not express these contrasts through the old dark/light color differentiation system, but the polarity is expressed by other means. A change in the scenes in which women are depicted may hold the answer to the question. Several scholars have noted that during the Classical period, as red figure becomes the dominant form of Athenian vase painting, there is a change toward images which either show women alone or place them in interior settings. As Lewis notes:

> Classical artists show women in far greater numbers than their early counterparts, but depict a much narrower range of themes, and these themes become stereotyping and inexpressive. Women are depicted almost exclusively in interior settings, in large or small groups, playing music, working wool or adorning themselves: images of domestic labour, of children and of sacrifice all become far less common. Some religious scenes still appear, for example the domestic festival of the Adonia, but we see much less of women outside the house.[51]

51. S. Lewis, *The Athenian Woman: An Iconographic Handbook* (London: Routledge, 2002), 130.

While color previously marked the ideological seclusion of women, now the repertoire of scenes differentiates between the male and female realm. This emphasis on women as secluded becomes the visual expression of the Athenian ideology of male/female difference.

During this period, costume also served to mark women as different. Lee's study of the revival of the peplos during the classical period describes the importance of that garment in constructing female gender in the fifth century. According to her analysis, the peplos brings together associations of women as both virtuous and treacherous fabric creators.[52] After all, women weave the peplos given to Athena, but they also wove the many killer cloaks of Greek mythology—Deianira's gift to Herakles and Medea's gift to Jason's new bride come readily to mind. As a heavy and confining garment, the peplos symbolized male control over the female body. Yet it is also suggests the multi-valent nature of women. Because of its construction (the sides are not fixed) it is also suitable for breast feeding. Thus, it marks the need to control women, but also the fact that they are nurturers and also bearers of legitimate offspring for the city.

Much scholarly attention has been devoted to determining the 'status' of women depicted in red figure. In particular, the question of whether women are "respectable" or paid companions is often raised. Scholars have searched, largely in vain, for status markers that would express this difference in types of women. Nudity was once thought to be a clear marker of lack of respectability for women. But while nude women shown at the symposium would seem to be paid companions, thorough studies of vase imagery have shown that there are situations in which even nude women are not prostitutes.[53]

The debate ranges not so much around images of nude women in symposium scenes, but rather women who are nude and engaging in seemingly domestic tasks such as spinning wool, as on a red-figure vase in Copenhagen[54] in which a nude female stands spinning in front of a clothed seated woman. Some have identified this scene, on the basis of the woman's nudity, as taking place in a brothel. Similarly vexing are scenes in which clothed women in domestic settings are approached by men holding sacks which are often identified as money

52. M. Lee, "Constructing Gender in the Feminine Greek Peplos," in L. Cleland, M. Harlow, and L. Llewellyn-Jones, *The Clothed Body in the Ancient World* (Oxford: Oxbow, 2005), 61–63.

53. S. Lewis, *The Athenian Woman*, 91–129.

54. Attic red-figure hydria, Cophenhagen National Museusm Chr. VIII; S. Lewis, *The Athenian Woman*, Fig. 3.10.

bags. Here the question is whether the women depicted are "housewives" getting the budget from their husbands or prostitutes receiving a client.[55] Despite many attempts, no clear-cut markers which would definitively identify these figures as one or the other have been successfully identified. This is a source of consternation to scholars seeking to use vases to reconstruct the lives of actual Athenian women. Examination of nude figures on vases has shown that, for women, nudity is not necessarily a reliable marker of whether a woman is part of the sex industry.

Ferrari suggests that we alter our viewpoint in respect to the much-debated red-figure vases. As she states:

> It is beside the point, therefore, to speculate whether in actuality courtesans worked wool or wives received gifts, because the fact that they did, if it were true, would not explain why they are represented doing so. The question to ask is what purposes it served to represent a woman (or girl) as both laborer and object of desire.[56]

Ferrari suggests that these images depict dual aspects of the same type of being. Like the image of woman presented by peplophoroi, vase-painting images can be read simultaneously in a variety of ways.

While in black figure the category 'woman' was clearly marked by color, a more nuanced expression of the qualities of the category woman is provided by

---

55. There is a huge bibliography on this topic. For the evolution of the discussion see among many others R. F. Sutton, Jr., *The Interaction Between Men and Women Portrayed on Attic Red-Figure Pottery* (Chapel Hill: University of North Carolina, 1981); D. Harvey, "Painted Ladies, Fact, Fiction and Fantasy," in *Proceedings of the 3rd Symposium on Ancient Greek and Related Pottery*, ed. J. Christiansen and T. Torben Melender (Copenhagen: Thorvaldsens Museum, 1988); C. Bérard, "The Order of Women," in *City of Images*, ed. C. Bérard et al. (Princeton: Princeton University Press, 1989); For men and money bags as a sign of prostitution see N. Hoesch, "Hetären," in *Kunstler Schale: Kultur des Trinkens*, ed. K. Vierneisel and B. Fellmann (Munich: Collection of Antiquities and Glyptothek, 1990), 228–34; For spinning hetaira as a prostitute see J. N. Davidson, *Courtesans and Fishcakes: The Consuming Passions of Classical Athens* (Chicago: University of Chicago Press, 1997); J. Neils, "Others Within the Other: an Intimate Look at Hetairai and Maeanads," in B. Cohen, *Not the Classical Ideal*, 203–26; U. Kreillinger, "To Be or Not to Be a Hetaira: Female Nudity in Classical Athens," in *Images and Gender: Contributions to the Hermeneutics of Reading Art*, ed. S. Schroer (Fribourg: Vandenhoeck & Ruprecht, 2006), 229–37; and K. M. Lynch, "Erotic Images on Attic Vases: Markets and Meanings," in *Markets and Meanings, Athenian Potters and Painters*, ed. J. Oakley and O. Palagia (Oxford: Oxford University Press, 2009). For a discussion of the evidence for prostitution in the Greek World, see A. Glazebrook and M. M. Henry, eds., *Greek Prostitutes in the Ancient Mediterranean 800 BCE–200 CE* (Madison: University of Wisconsin Press, 2011).
56. G. Ferrari, *Figures of Speech: Men and Maidens in Ancient Greece* (Chicago: University of Chicago Press, 2002), 21.

red figure. Rather than marking women as different by color, they are marked by setting and sphere of activity as different. And within that category of difference, aspects of their nature are explored through the much-debated images of such figures as the "spinning hetaera." The lack of male/female color differentiation in red figure combined with the new interest in interior scenes is perfectly in keeping with the mores of Athenian society in which the ideological role of woman, no matter what her actual role, was as an interior, secluded, and fundamentally different role from that of man. The difference includes a nature that can be expressed as both chaste and wild, as wife and hetaira.

Thus we can see that although red figure no longer depicts tan men and pale women, the ideas of fundamental female difference which lay behind this earlier method of distinction are certainly not abandoned. Instead, they are simply expressed differently. In the face of foreign threats, solidarity of form (everyone the same color) is privileged over male/female color differentiation and differences are expressed by theme rather than by color. Costume and setting give subtle clues about women's role. Without the startlingly visual contrast, a more nuanced but equally polarized depiction of women becomes the norm. As with black-figure images, we are here dealing with a constructed reality. Because its images are more naturalistic, red figure may seduce us into believing that we are looking at more realistic views of the actual lives of women, but the scenes are no more realistic than those presented with sharp color distinction between male and female in black figure.

Red figure's abandonment of male/female color differentiation is anomalous when placed against other media. We should remember also that color continues to be a defining mark of difference in the theater, where female masks are white, and also possibly in wall painting. Again, preserved ancient Athenian wall painting is lacking, but white-ground vases produced during this period may give a suggestion of the color palettes employed, since the white background of these vases is generally considered to be analogous to the blank background of a wall painting. As Mertens notes, the white rather than orange clay surface helped to link vase painting with wall painting, a significant medium after the Persian Wars.[57] As discussed above, during the Late Archaic experimental period when red figure was developed, white-ground vases used outline drawing. In keeping with the common skin color used for men and women in red figure, both male and female were left the color of the background. Around

57. J. R. Mertens, "Attic White Ground: Potter and Painter," in *The Colors of Clay*, 189.

470 BC these vases show a short-lived experiment in which an additional layer of a brighter, white paint is used for female flesh.[58] This is eventually abandoned. Wehgartner suggests that this may be because this brighter white for women had the unintended consequence of emphasizing the fact that men's flesh was white (cream rather than bright white) as well.[59] The fact that female flesh was emphasized initially rather than male suggests that white ground is responding to the anxiety about women during this period which we have mentioned earlier. Around 450 BC white ground became perhaps even more consonant with wall painting through the use of matt colors applied after firing and a lighter and more porous background.[60]

Men are now painted a dark brown color and women left the color of the background. This feature may be connected to wall painting, which again is unfortunately not preserved. It is, however, tempting to see this renewed emphasis on color/gender distinctions as a reflection of the importance placed on Athenian women by Perikles' citizenship law, which required that both parents had to be 'native Athenians' for a male to hold citizenship.[61] This period also corresponds to a marked increase in popularity of white-ground funerary lekythoi. Neils suggests that since funerary ritual was the prerogative of women, the white ground is also symbolic of the traditional white color used for women.[62]

Of course the question remains as to why red figure did not re-institute male/female color differentiation. The answer may lie in the color palettes available to white-ground painters vs. those available to red-figure painters. White ground always had the potential to be a more polychrome medium, since the white background was similar to that of wall and panel painting which used a varied palette. This connection with wall painting appears in particular in an exceptional and late group (c. 400 BC) of five large lekythoi attributed to Athens and grouped under the name "Huge Lekythoi."[63]These seem to have been designed not as containers but rather as grave markers, so they may also indicate a possible color palette for sculpture as well since they fill the same role as grave stelai. Male/female color differentiation is firmly in place. Men's flesh is

58. J. H. Oakley, *Picturing Death in Classical Athens*, 6–7.
59. I. Wehgartner, *Attische weisgrunde Keramik*, 26.
60. J. R. Mertens, "Attic White Ground: Potter and Painter," in *The Colors of Clay*, 191.
61. For prominence of Amazons reflecting Perikles' legislation see Stewart, "Imag(in)ing the Other," 571–97.
62. J. Neils, "Women are White: White Ground and the Attic Funeral," in *Papers on Special Techniques in Athenian Vases* (Los Angeles: Getty Museum, 2008), 203–26.
63. M. Robertson, *The Art of Vase Painting in Classical Athens*, 254. J. R. Mertens, "Attic White Ground: Potter and Painter," Cat. Nos. 68 and 69.

painted a dark brown and women's added white. A close connection to wall painting is suggested by these vases' employment of one of the techniques which ancient sources tell us was being perfected by wall painters at this time, namely the use of shading to suggest dimensionality. Here, however, the male/female dichotomy is further emphasized, since shading is used only for the flesh of men, not women.[64] The diversion between red-figure and white-ground/panel painting suggests that red figure remains primarily a vase-painting technique and does not fully partake of the developments of monumental painting.

Red figure's lack of male/female color differentiation is not uniform during the late Classical period. In the 420s, in particular, vases become more decorative with the addition of added clay and in some instances added white. The Medias Painter is one of the main proponents of the more ornate style.[65] White, however, is not consistently used to depict female flesh. On a squat lekythos attributed to the Painter of the Frankfort Acorn, the lone male figure is left the reserve color of the clay, and all of the female figures are painted white, but the Erotes are also painted white.[66] Several other vases provide examples of this inconsistency. On a pyxis in Oxford showing women and Erotes in a garden, only the Erotes are painted white.[67] A Volute crater by the Pronomos Painter depicting Dionysos and a gathering of actors and Herakles is a tour de force of the variety of ways in which added white can be used.[68] As such it also shows the inconsistency with which male/female color differentiation can be applied during this period. White is used for the flesh of Ariadne and for one of the presumably female theater masks, but it is also used for the bearded male masks carried by Herakles and one of the actors. The breastplate of Herakles and the shaggy costume of one of the satyr play actors are also highlighted with white. White accents serve to highlight the main figures. A mid-fourth century pelike by the Marsyas Painter combines white for female flesh with white for emphasis.[69] Peleus and Thetis are shown wrestling surrounded by nymphs and Eros.

64. M. Robertson, *The Art of Vase Painting in Classical Athens*, 254.
65. See L. Burn, *The Meidias Painter* (Oxford, Clarendon Press, 1987).
66. Malibu, J. Paul Getty Museum. AE 10. Beazley, J. D. *Attic Red-Figure Vase Painters*. 2nd edition. (Oxford: Clarendon Press, 1963) 1313.3. B. Cohen, *Colors of Clay*, No. 34, p. 133.
67. L. Burn, *The Meidias Painter*, M 29.
68. Naples 3240 J.D Beazley,*Attic Red-Figure Vase Painters* (Oxford: Clarendon Press, 1942).1336.1, J. Boardman, *Athenian Red-figure Vases, the Classical Period* (New York: Thames and Hudson, 1998), 323.
69. London E. 424 from Camirus, J. D. Beazley, *Attic Red-Figure Vase Painters* (Oxford: Clarendon Press, 1942). 1475.4. J. Boardman, *Athenian Red-figure Vases, the Classical Period*, 390.

Only Thetis and Eros are painted white and while white is certainly appropriate for Thetis, it would be equally appropriate for the nymphs who are left the reserved color of the clay. Instead, white serves as a kind of spotlight drawing attention to Thetis and Eros. Thus while male/female color differentiation remains consonant with many underlying ideas about women, and added white for female flesh could be seen as a perhaps as a nod toward traditionalism during troubled times, its inconsistent use suggests that decorative concerns outweigh gender messages. This use of white as a highlighting device could also be a response to the increasing sophistication of wall painting in which shadows and shading are being employed. The last truly Athenian red-figure style, seen in Kerch vases, continues this use of white sometimes for gender and sometimes for highlighting.[70]

As Athenian fortunes begin to wane with disastrous military defeats, South Italian vase painting becomes the dominant form. Here white is sometimes added for female flesh, but not exclusively. It can also be used to indicate the deceased in funerary scenes. Funerary naiskoi are popular subject matter and the figure standing within them, presumably the deceased or a statue of the deceased, is painted white regardless of gender.[71]

We return again to the questions posed at the beginning of this chapter. As seen in the reigns of Hatshepsut and Akhenaten, does the change in male/female color differentiation found in red figure coincide with a change in ideology or is something else at work? We have seen that several factors, both ideological and artistic, influenced this change in style. Lack of male/female color differentiation may be consonant with the newly emphasized polarity of Athenian versus foreigner. The ability to draw more detailed distinctions of clothing and physiognomy provided by the new technique made this possible without abandoning the gender ideas which had shaped earlier Athenian society. Gender anxieties could be expressed in a more nuanced way through the choice of scene and theme depicted, to the point that added white flesh can serve a decorative and emphatic function rather than its previous role in gender distinction. However, just as in Egyptian art, when we look at images of women on red-figure vases we are not looking at actual lives of women but of the gender constructs which dominated Athenian society.

---

70. K. Lapatin, "Kerch Style Vases," in B. Cohen, ed., *Colors of Clay*, 317–41.

71. For examples see M. Mayo, ed., *The Art of South Italy: Vases from Magna Graecia* (Richmond: Virginia Museum of Fine Arts, 1982), and J. G. Pedley, *Greek Art and Archaeology*, 9.47 and 9.51.

Conclusion

I began this study by asking a number of questions. First and foremost was whether the designation in Attic black figure of males as dark and women as light had any underlying significance. My answer to that question is a resounding "Yes." Color expressed underlying polarization of male and female that was a key organizing principle of ancient Athenian society. While previously dismissed as simply a convention of ancient art, male/female color differentiation in fact provides an important tool for understanding gender relations. Such a commonplace phenomenon proved to be a complex and multivalent method for expressing ideas about the relationship between men and women, a method flexible enough to encompass several world views. Egypt's long tradition of male/female color differentiation was based on Egyptian ideas about the place of male and female in the correct ordering of the universe and on ideologies of power connected to the role of pharaoh. Its absence proved as significant as its presence. In Athens the use of male/female color differentiation shows the fundamental underlying message that women are a distinct species from men. In those periods in both parts of the ancient world when color differentiation was not employed—the reigns of the Egyptian pharaohs Hatshepsut and Akhenaten, and the Classical period in Athens—change reflected changed ideology and/or a different expression of the same ideology.

When we compare Egypt and Greece we see that the use of color to distinguish between male and female has a complex history. The same basic pattern, dark men and light women, can, as in Egypt, symbolize reconcilable opposites and, as in Greece, symbolize seemingly irreconcilable opposites. What in Egypt expressed the unity of male and female in Greece expressed polarity. Comparing Greece and Egypt revealed that something considered a simple convention is much more complicated. In ancient Egypt nuances of power, especially the establishment of pharaonic rule and theology, combined in the "establishment of the norm" of male/female color differentiation.

Different factors led to the use of the same visual code in Greece. While gender was always an underlying organizing principle of Greek art, the dark/light expression of difference came to the fore during the Orientalizing period. Hesiod and Homer are the literary expressions of this ideal. The increased Greek presence in Egypt allowed the Greeks to see painting and sculpture that used this system, but it was the fact that these visual statements of gender difference resonated with their own underlying ideology that caused them to be adopted. It was not necessary for Greeks to understand or even to accept the Egyptian point of view to find their method of representation a usable feature. Male/female color differentiation became a *calque*, a loan followed by translation into a native idiom.[1] The transformation occurs in the emphasis on a sharper color contrast in Greece than in Egypt. While yellow could also be used for female flesh in Egypt, because it was an oppositional color to red, Greek art prefers the sharper polarity expressed through the contrast of white for female flesh. Thus, the same stylistic feature can express different things in different societies and should be looked at on a case-by-case basis. Even within the Greek world the differences between Athens and Corinth, for example, in the use of color shows color used to express on the one hand sharp gender distinctions/gender polarities and on the other to provide a decorative and pleasing pattern.

However, an understanding of the artistic expression of this ideology has been missing from the scholarly literature for a number of reasons. One is that Greek experiments with perfecting the human form, culminating in the Classical ideal preserved in such monuments as the Parthenon sculptures, have caused us to overlook the fact that something besides the pursuit of naturalism was involved in Greek art. The lack of preserved monumental wall painting from ancient Greece, combined with the tantalizing descriptions of technical advances in the portrayal of figures in space that Pliny gives us in reference to the lost works of ancient Greek painters, has kept attention away from the more symbolic aspects of Greek art. In addition, the understandable desire on the part of scholars to find some traces of everyday life in the multitudinous images preserved on Greek vases has shifted the focus away from analysis of such a

1. S. Morris, *Daidalos and the Origins of Greek Art* (Princeton: Princeton University Press, 1992), 98.

seemingly mundane feature as the use of color to differentiate figures. Such symbolism is usually considered the province of Egyptian art, with its supposedly formulaic figures. Formulaic features of Archaic art are overlooked as bumps on the way to the development of the Classical ideal.

Pollock states that "ideology cannot be divorced from power relations, but in contrast to domination, which depends on coercion, ideology works by winning consent. The consent is not to the underlying goals, but rather to the superficial aspects of the ideology which produces a world view that comes to seem 'natural' or 'common sense.'"[2] By overlooking male/female color differentiation we have been unwitting participants in accepting this world view. I hope my study has revealed the need to look beyond the surface for a deeper understanding of the underpinnings of traditional artistic forms. As I have shown, the answer to the question of underlying meaning for what at first seems to be the identical form is not always the same.

One of the troubles with such a wide-ranging study is that everyone can attack a section based on his or her own field of expertise. However, I think we do our field a disservice by not attempting to look at the big picture. We are reminded in each instance that what we are dealing with in art is not everyday reality but a conceptual view of ideal relationships based on each society's world view. More work remains to be done. Other ancient societies also used male/female color differentiation. Do Etruscans follow this practice because they imitate Greek forms or commission Greek artists to decorate their tombs with paintings? Or is something more at work? Do the Romans simply follow Greek practice? Specific study of both of these groups may yield a more nuanced understanding of their gender ideology, but that must await another book.

---

2. S. Pollock, *Ancient Mesopotamia: The Eden that Never Was* (Cambridge: Cambridge University Press, 1999), 175.

Bibliography

Adams, B., and K. M. Cialowicz. *Protodynastic Egypt*. Buckinghamshire: Shire Publications, 1997.

Aldred, C. *Akhenaten and Nefertiti*. New York: Brooklyn Museum/Viking Press, 1973.

Alexandridou, A. *The Early Black-figured Pottery of Attika in Context (c. 630–570 BCE)*. Leiden: Brill, 2011.

Aloupi-Siotis, E. "Discovery and Revival of Attic Vase Decoration Techniques: What Can They Offer Archaeological Research?" In *Papers on Special Techniques in Athenian Vases*, edited by K. Lapatin, 113–28. Los Angeles: J. Paul Getty Museum, 2008.

Amyx, D. A. *Corinthian Vase-painting of the Archaic Period*. Berkeley: University of California Press, 1988.

Antonaccio, C. M. "Contesting the Past: Hero Cult, Tomb Cults and Epic in Early Greece." *American Journal of Archaeology* 98, No. 3 (1994): 389–410.

Arnold, Dieter. "The Temple of Hatshepsut at Deir el-Bahri." In *Hatshepsut from Queen to Pharaoh*, edited by C. H. Roehrig, R. Dreyfus, and C. Keller, 135–40. New York: Metropolitan Museum of Art, 2005.

Arnold, Dorothea. "Aspects of the Royal Female Image." In *The Royal Women of Amarna*, 85–93. New York: Metropolitan Museum of Art, 1997.

Arnold, Dorothea. *When the Pyramids Were Built: Egyptian Art of the Old Kingdom*. New York: Rizzoli International Publications, 1999.

Arnold, D., L. Green, and J. Allen, eds. *The Royal Women of Amarna: Aspects of Beauty from Ancient Egypt*. New York: Metropolitan Museum of Art, 1997.

Arnold, D., K. Grzymski, and C. Ziegler. *Egyptian Art in the Age of the Pyramids*. New York: Metropolitan Museum of Art, 1999.

Arnold, D., K. Grzymski, and C. Ziegler. "The Destruction of the Statues of Hatshepsut from Deir el-Bahri." In *Hatshepsut from Queen to Pharaoh*, edited by C. H. Roehrig, 270–76. New York: Metropolitan Museum of Art, 2005.

Asher-Greve, J. M. "The Essential Body: Mesopotamian Conceptions of the Gendered Body." In *Gender and the Body in the Ancient Mediterranean*, edited by M. Wyke, 8–37. Oxford: Blackwell Publishers, 1998.

Bahrani, Z. *Women of Babylon: Gender and Representation in Mesopotamia*. London: Routledge, 2001.

Baines, J. "Color Terminology and Color Classification: Ancient Egyptian Color Terminology and Polychromy." *American Anthropologist* 87 (1985): 282–97.

Baines, J. *Fecundity Figures: Egyptian Personification and the Iconology of a Genre*. Chicago: Griffith Institute, 1985.

Baines, J. *Visual and Written Culture in Ancient Egypt*. New York: Oxford University Press, 2009.

Beazley, J. D. *Attic Red-Figure Vase-Painters*. 1942. 2nd edition. Oxford: Clarendon Press, 1963.

Beazley, J. D. *Paralipomena: Additions to Attic Black-figure Vase-painters and to Attic Red-figure Vase-painters*. 2nd edition. Oxford: Oxford University Press, 1971.

Beazley, J. D. *Attic Black-Figure Vase-Painters*. New York: Hacker Art Books, 1978.

Benson, J. L. *Horse, Bird and Man*. Amherst: University of Massachusetts Press, 1970.

Bérard, C. "The Order of Women." In *A City of Images: Iconography and Society in Ancient Greece*, edited by C. Bérard, C. Bron, J-L. Durand, F. Frontisi-Ducroux, A. Lissarrague, A. Schnapp, and J. P. Vernant, 89–108. Princeton: Princeton University Press, 1989.

Bérard, C. "The Image of the Other and the Foreign Hero." In *Not the Classical Ideal: Athens and the Construction of the Other in Greek Art*, edited by B. Cohen, 390–412. Leiden: Brill Academic Publishers, 2000.

Berlin, B., and P. Kay. *Basic Color Terms: Their Universality and Evolution*. Berkeley: University of California Press, 1969.

Bernal, M. *Black Athena: The Afro-Asiatic Roots of Classical Civilization*. New Brunswick: Rutgers, 1987.

Bianchi, R. *Splendors of Ancient Egypt*. London: Booth-Clibborn, 1996.

Boardman, J. *Athenian Black Figure Vases*. London: Thames and Hudson, 1974.

Boardman, J. *The Greeks Overseas*. London: Thames and Hudson, 1980.

Boardman, J. *Greek Art*. London: Thames and Hudson, 1985.

Boardman, J. *Athenian Red Figure Vases: The Archaic Period*. London: Thames and Hudson, 1985.

Boardman, J. *Pre-Classical: From Crete to Archaic Greece*. Baltimore: Penguin, 1997.

Boardman, J. *Early Greek Vase Painting: 11th–6th Centuries BC*. London: Thames and Hudson, 1998.

Boardman, J. *The History of Greek Vases: Potters, Painters and Pictures*. London: Thames and Hudson, 2001.

Breasted, J. H. *The Conquest of Civilization*. New York: HarperCollins, 1926 (revised 1938).

Breasted, J. H. *Egyptian Servant Statues*. New York: Pantheon Books, 1948.
Brinkmann, V. *Beobachtungen zum formalin Aufbau und zum Sinngehalt der Friese des Siphnierschatzhauses*. Munich: Ennepetal, 1994.
Brinkmann, V. "Die Polychromie der Archaischen und Frühklassischen Skulptur." In *Studien zur Antiken Malerei und Farbgebung* 5, edited by R. Biering and V. Brinkmann. Munich: Biering & Brinkmann, 2003.
Brinkmann, V. *Die Polychromie der Archaischen und Frühklassischen Skulptur*. Munich: Biering & Brinkmann, 2003.
Brinkmann, V. "Die Farben der Archaischen und Frühklassischen Skulptur." In *Bunte Götter, Die Farbigkeit Antike Skulptur*, edited by V. Brinkmann, 35–83. Munich: Biering & Brinkmann, 2004.
Brown, S. "'Ways of Seeing' Women in Antiquity: An Introduction to Feminism in Classical Art and Archaeology." In *Naked Truths: Women, Sexuality and Gender in Classical Art and Archaeology*, edited by A. O. Koloski-Ostrow and C. L. Lyons, 14–18. London: Routledge, 1997.
Bruno, V. J. *Form and Color in Greek Painting*. New York: Norton, 1977.
Bryan, B. "In Women Good and Bad Fortune Are on Earth: Status and Roles of Women in Egyptian Culture." In *Mistress of the House, Mistress of Heaven: Women in Ancient Egypt*, edited by A. Capel and G. Markoe, 25–46. New York: Hudson Hills Press, 1996.
Burkert, W. *The Orientalizing Revolution: Near Eastern Influence in the Early Archaic Age*. Cambridge: Harvard University Press, 1992.
Burn, L. *The Meidias Painter*. Oxford: Clarendon Press, 1987.
Caminos, R. A. 1988. *Semna-Kumma, Vol. 1: The Temple of Semna, Archaeological Survey of Egypt*, 37th Memoir. London: Egypt Exploration Society, 1988.
Capel, A. "Goddesses: Catalogue Entry 53a and b." In *Mistress of the House, Mistress of Heaven: Women in Ancient Egypt*, edited by A. Capel and G. Markoe, 121–22. New York: Hudson Hills Press, 1996.
Capel, A., and G. Markoe, eds. *Mistress of the House, Mistress of Heaven: Women in Ancient Egypt*. New York: Hudson Hills Press, 1996.
Carter, J. A., and L. J. Steinburg. "Kouroi and Statistics." *American Journal of Archaeology* 114 (2010): 103–28.
Case, H., and J. C. Payne. "Tomb 100: The Decorated Tomb at Hierakonpolis." *Journal of Egyptian Archaeology* 48 (1962): 5–18.
Chapin, A. P., ed. *ΧΑΡΙΣ: Essays in Honor of Sara A. Immerwahr*. Princeton: American School of Classical Studies, 2004.
Cheal, C. "The Meaning of Skin Color in Eighteenth Dynasty Egypt." In *Race and Identity in the Nile Valley*, edited by C. Fluehr-Lobban and K. Rhodes, 47–70. Trenton, NJ: Red Sea Press.
Cherpion, N. "The Human Image in Old Kingdom Nonroyal Reliefs." In *Egyptian Art in the Age of the Pyramids*, edited by D. Arnold, K. Gryzmski, and C. Ziegler, 103–16. New York: Metropolitan Museum of Art, 1999.

Chevrier, H. "Rapport sur les travaux de Karnak." *Annales du Service des Antiquités de l'Égypt* (March–May 1926): 119–30.

Chevrier, H. "Rapport sur les travaux de Karnak." *Annales du Service des Antiquités de l'Égypt* 34 (1933–34): 159–76.

Cialowicz, K. M. "Pre-dynastic Period." In *The Oxford Encyclopedia of Ancient Egypt*, Vol. 3, edited by D. B. Redford, 61–65. Oxford: Oxford University Press, 2001.

Cleland, L. "The Semiosis of Description: Some Research on Fabric and Colour in the Brauron Inventories." In *The Clothed Body in the Ancient World*, edited by L. Cleland, M. Harlow, and L. Llewellyn-Jones, 87–95. Oxford: Oxbow Books, 2005.

Cleland, L., and K. Stears, eds. *Colour in the Ancient Mediterranean World.*, BAR International Series 1267. Oxford: *British Archaeological Reports*, 2004.

Cline, E. H. *Sailing the Wine-Dark Sea: International Trade and the Late Bronze Age Aegean.* Oxford: *British Archaeological Reports*, 1994.

Cohen, B., ed. *Not the Classical Ideal: Athens and the Construction of the Other in Greek Art.* Leiden: Brill Academic Publishers, 2000.

Cohen, B., ed. *The Colors of Clay: Special Techniques in Athenian Vases.* Los Angeles: J. Paul Getty Museum, 2006.

Cohen, B. "Six's Technique: Black Ground." In *The Colors of Clay: Special Techniques in Athenian Vases*, edited by B. Cohen, 72–104. Los Angeles: J. Paul Getty Museum, 2006.

Cohen, B. "Bilingual Vases and Vase-Painters." In *The Colors of Clay: Special Techniques in Athenian Vases*, edited by B. Cohen, 17–42. Los Angeles: J. Paul Getty Museum, 2006.

Cohen, B. "Outline in Black- and Red-Figure Vase-Painting: Outline as a Special Technique in Black- and Red-figure Vase-painting." In *The Colors of Clay*, edited by B. Cohen, 149–61. Los Angeles: J. Paul Getty Museum, 2006.

Coldstream, J. N. "The Geometric Style: Birth of the Picture." In *Looking at Greek Vases*, edited by T. Rasmussen and N. Spivey, 37–56. Cambridge: Cambridge University Press, 1991.

Coleman, J. E., and C. A. Walt, eds. *Greeks and Barbarians: Essays on Interactions between Greeks and Non-Greeks in Antiquity and the Consequences for Eurocentrism.* Bethesda, MD: CDL Press, 1997.

Collon, D. *Ancient Near Eastern Art.* Berkeley: University of California Press, 1995.

Connelly, J. B. *Portrait of a Priestess: Women and Ritual.* Princeton: Princeton University Press, 2007.

Cook, R. M. "Fikellura Pottery." *Annual of the British School at Athens* 34 (1933–34): 1–98.

Cook, R. M. "A List of Clazomenian Pottery." *Annual of the British School at Athens* 47 (1952): 123–52.

Corner, S. "Bringing the Outside In: The *Andrōn* as Brothel and the Symposium's Civic Sexuality." In *Greek Prostitutes in the Ancient Mediterranean, 800 BCE–200 CE*, edited by A. Glazebrook and M. Henry, 60–85. Madison: University of Wisconsin Press, 2011.

Davidson, J. N. *Courtesans and Fishcakes: The Consuming Passions of Classical Athens.* Chicago: University of Chicago Press, 1997.

Davies, W. W., ed. *Colour and Painting in Ancient Egypt.* London: British Museum Press, 2001.

Dean-Jones, L. *Women's Bodies in Classical Greek Science.* Oxford: Oxford University Press, 1994.

Dean-Jones, L. "The Cultural Construct of the Female Body in Classical Greek Science." In *Sex and Difference in Ancient Greece and Rome*, edited by M. Golden and P. Toohey, 183–201. Edinburgh: Edinburgh University Press, 2003. Originally printed in *Women's History and Ancient History*, edited by S. B. Pomeroy, 111–37. Chapel Hill: University of North Carolina Press, 1991.

Diop, C. A. *The African Origins of Civilization.* Chicago: Lawrence Hill Books, 1974.

Dorman, F. "Hatshepsut: Princess to Queen to Co-Ruler." In *Hatshepsut from Queen to Pharaoh*, edited by C. H. Roehrig, 87–90. New York: Metropolitan Museum of Art, 2005.

Dorman, F. "The Destruction of Hatshepsut's Memory: The Proscription of Hatshepsut." In *Hatshepsut from Queen to Pharaoh*, edited by C. H. Roehrig, 270–76. New York: Metropolitan Museum of Art, 2005.

Eaverly, M. A. "Color and Gender in Ancient Painting: A Pan-Mediterranean Approach." In *From the Ground Up: Beyond Gender Theory in Archaeology*, edited by N. Wicker and Bettina Arnold, 5–10. BAR International Series, 812. Oxford: British Archaeological Reports, 1999.

Eaverly, M. A. "The Iconography of Gender: Dark Men and Light Women in Archaic Painting." In *Common Ground: Archaeology, Art, Science and the Humanities*, edited by C. C. Mattusch, A. A. Donahue, and A. Brauer, 488–90. Proceedings of the XVI International Congress of Classical Archaeology. Oxford: Oxbow Books, 2003.

Eaverly, M. A. "Colors of Power, Brown Men and Brown Women in the Art of Akhenaten." In *Colour in the Ancient Mediterranean World*, edited by L. Cleland and K. Stears, 53–55. BAR International Series, 1267. Oxford: British Archaeological Reports, 2004.

Eaverly, M. A. "Dark Men, Light Women: Origins of Color as Gender Indicator in Ancient Egypt." In *The World of Women in the Ancient and Classical Near East*, edited by B. Nakhai, 1–12. London: Cambridge Scholars Publishing, 2008.

Erman, A. *Ancient Egyptian Poetry and Prose.* Translated by Alyward Blackman. New York: Dover, 1995. First published 1923.

Evans, A. *The Palace of Minos.* Vol. I. London: Macmillan, 1921.

Fathom, E. *Women in the Classical World: Image and Text.* New York: Oxford University Press, 1994.

Faulkner, R. O. *The Ancient Egyptian Pyramid Texts.* Oxford: Oxford University Press, 1969.

Ferrari, G. "Menelās." *Journal of Hellenic Studies* 107 (1987): 180–82.

Ferrari, G. *Figures of Speech, Men and Maidens in Ancient Greece*. Chicago: University of Chicago Press, 2002.

Filipzak, Z. *Hot Dry Men, Cold Wet Women: The Theory of Humors in Western European Art, 1575–1700*. New York: American Federation of Arts, 1997.

Fischer, H. G. "Varia Aegyptiaca 1. Yellow-Skinned Representations of Men in the Old Kingdom." *Journal of the American Research Center in Egypt* 2 (1963): 17–22.

Fischer, H. G. *Egyptian Women of the Old Kingdom and of the Heracleopolitan Period*. New York: Metropolitan Museum of Art, 1989.

Frandsen, P. J. "On Categorization and Metaphorical Structuring: Some Remarks on Egyptian Art and Language." *Cambridge Archaeological Journal* 7, No. 1 (1977): 71–104.

Freed, R. E., Y. J. Markowitz, and S. H. D'Auria, eds. *Pharaohs of the Sun*. Boston: Bulfinch Press, 1999.

Freed, R. E. "Art in the Service of Religion and State." In *Pharaohs of the Sun*, edited by R. E. Freed, Y. J. Markowitz, and S. H. D'Auria, 110–30. Boston: Bulfinch Press, 1999.

Freed, R. E. "Art." In *The Oxford Encyclopedia of Ancient Egypt*, Vol. 1, edited by D. B. Redford, 127–36. Oxford: Oxford University Press, 2001.

Gage, J. *Color and Culture*. Little, Brown. Boston, 1993.

Gage, J. *Color and Meaning, Art, Science,and Symbolism*. Berkeley: University of California Press, 1999.

Gardiner, A. H., T. E. Peet, and J. Ĉerný. *The Inscriptions of Sinai*. Oxford: Egypt Exploration Society, 1952–55.

Gates, C. "The Adoption of Pictorial Imagery in Minoan Painting: A Comparativist Perspective." In *ΧΑΡΙΣ: Essays in Honor of Sara A. Immerwahr*. Hesperia Supplement 33, edited by A. P. Chapin, 27–46.Princeton: American School of Classical Studies, 2004.

Gero, J. M., and M. W. Conkey, eds. *Engendering Archaeology, Women and Prehistory*. London: Wiley-Blackwell, 1991.

Gilbert, P. "Les sens des portraits intacts de Hatshepsout à Deir el-Bhari." *Chronique d'Egypte*, No. 56 (1953): 219–22.

Gillam, R. A. "Sobekneferu." In *The Oxford Encyclopedia of Ancient Egypt*, edited by D. B. Redford, 301. Oxford: Oxford University Press, 2001.

Glazebrook, H., and M. M. Henry, eds. *Greek Prostitutes in the Ancient Mediterranean, 800 BCE–200 CE*. Madison: University of Wisconsin Press, 2011.

Golden, M., and P. Toohey, eds. *Sex and Difference in Ancient Greece and Rome*. Edinburgh: Edinburgh University Press, 2003.

Gombrich, E. H. *Art and Illusion: A Study in the Psychology of Pictorial Representation*. Baltimore: Johns Hopkins University Press, 1977.

Goodison, L., and C. Morris, eds. *Ancient Goddesses, The Myths and the Evidence*. London: British Museum Press, 1998.

Goodman, N. *Languages of Art*. Indianapolis: Hackett Publishing, 1976.

Gould, J. "Law, Custom and Myth: Aspects of the Social Position of Women in Classical Athens." *Journal of Hellenic Studies* 100 (1980): 38–59.

Grzymski, K. "Royal Statuary." In *Egyptian Art in the Age of the Pyramids*, edited by D. Arnold and C. Ziegler, 51–56. New York: Metropolitan Museum of Art, 1999.

Gunter, A. C. *Greek Art and the Orient*. Cambridge: Cambridge University Press, 2009.

Guralnick, E. "The Egyptian Greek Connection in the 8th to 6th Centuries BC: An Overview." In *Greeks and Barbarians: Essays on Interactions between Greeks and Non-Greeks in Antiquity and the Consequences for Eurocentrism*, edited by J. E. Coleman and C. A. Walt, 127–54. Bethesda, MD: CDL Press, 1997.

Habachi, L. "Two Graffitti at Sehēl from the Reign of Queen Hatshepsut." *Journal of Near Eastern Studies* 16 (April 1957): 88–104.

Harari, I. "Nature de la stele de donation de fonction du roi Ahmosis à la reine Ahmês Nefertari." *Annales du Service des Antiquités de l'Égypt* 56 (1959): 139–201.

Hardin, C. L., and L. Maffi, eds. *Color Categories in Thought and Language*. Cambridge: Cambridge University Press, 1997.

Hartwig, B. K. "Painting." In *The Oxford Encyclopedia of Ancient Egypt*, Vol. 3, edited by D. B. Redford, 1–12. Oxford: Oxford University Press, 2001.

Harvey, D. "Painted Ladies, Fact, Fiction and Fantasy." In *Proceedings of the 3rd Symposium on Ancient Greek and Related Pottery*, edited by J. Christiansen and T. Torben Melender, 242–57. Copenhagen: Thorvaldsens Museum, 1988.

Hassan, F. "Earliest Goddesses of Egypt: Divine Mothers and Cosmic Bodies." In *Ancient Goddesses: The Myths and the Evidence*, edited by B. Goodison and C. Morris, 98–112. Madison: University of Wisconsin Press, 1998.

Hassan, F. "Primeval Goddess to Divine King: The Mythogenesis of Power in the Early Egyptian State." In *The Followers of Horus: Studies Dedicated to Michael Allen Hoffman*, edited by R. Friedman and B. Adams, 307–21. Oxford: Egyptian Studies Publications, 1992.

Hawass, Z. *Silent Images: Women in Pharaonic Egypt*. New York: America University in Cairo Press, 1999.

Hawass, Z. *The Royal Tombs of Egypt: The Art of Thebes Revealed*. London: Thames and Hudson, 2006.

Hemelrijk, J. M. *Caeretan Hydriae*. Mainz am Rhein: Zabern, 1984.

Henderson, J. "Smashing Bodies: The Corinthian Tydeus and Ismene Amphora (Louvre E640)." In *Constructions of the Classical Body*, edited by J. I. Porter, 19–49. Ann Arbor: University of Michigan Press, 1999.

Higgins, R. *Minoan and Mycenaean Art*. London: Thames and Hudson, 1967.

Hill, M. "Dwarf Musician." In *Egyptian Art in the Age of the Pyramids*, edited by D. Arnold, C. Ziegler, and C. Roehrig, 391. New York: Metropolitan Museum of Art, 1999.

Hiller, F., and K. Braun, and A. E. Furtwängler eds. *Studien Zur Klassischen Archäologie, Festschrift für Friedrich Hiller zu seinem 60.Geburstag am 12 März 1986*. Saarbrücken: Amsterdam Archaeological Institute of the Saarland University, 1986.

Hoesch, N. "Hetären." In *Kunstler Schale: Kultur des Trinkens*, edited by K. Vierneisel and B. Fellmann, 228–34. Munich: Collection of Antiquities and Glyptothek, 1990.

Hoffman, G. *Imports and Immigrants: Near Eastern Contacts with Iron Age Crete.* Ann Arbor: University of Michigan Press, 1997.

Hurwit, J. M. *The Art and Culture of Early Greece, 1100–480 B.C.* Ithaca: Cornell University Press, 1985.

Hurwit, J. M. "Art, Poetry and the Polis in the Age of Homer." In *From Pasture to Polis: Art in the Age of Homer*, edited by S. Langdon, 14–42. Columbia: University of Missouri Press, 1993.

Hurwit, J. M. "Beautiful Evil: Pandora and the Athena Parthenos." *American Journal of Archaeology* 99, No. 2 (1995): 171–86.

Hurwit, J. M. *The Athenian Acropolis.* Cambridge: Cambridge University Press, 2000.

Hurwit, J. M. "Reading the Chigi Vase." *Hesperia* 71, No. 1 (2002): 1–22.

Immerwahr, S. A. *Aegean Painting in the Bronze Age.* University Park: Pennsylvania State University Press, 1990.

Irwin, E. *Colour Terms in Greek Poetry.* Toronto: Edgar Kent, 1974.

Isaac, B. *The Invention of Racism in Classical Antiquity.* Princeton: Princeton University Press, 2004.

Jenkins, I., and V. Turner. *The Greek Body.* Los Angeles: J. Paul Getty Museum, 2009.

Johnson, J. "The Legal Status of Women in Ancient Egypt." In *Mistress of the House, Mistress of Heaven: Women in Ancient Egypt*, edited by A. K. Capel and G. E. Markoe, 175–86. New York: Hudson Hill Press, 1996.

Johnson, W. R. "The Setting: History, Religion and Art." In *Pharaohs of the Sun*, edited by R. Freed, Y. Markowitz, and S. D'Auria, 38–49. London: Thames and Hudson, 1999.

Jones, L. D. "The Classical Construct of the Female Body in Classical Greek Science." In *Women's History and Ancient History*, edited by S. B. Pomeroy, 110–37. Chapel Hill: University of North Carolina Press, 1991.

Just, R. *Women in Athenian Law and Life.* London: Routledge, 1989.

Kampen, N. B., ed. *Sexuality in Ancient Art.* Cambridge: Cambridge University Press, 1996.

Keesling, C. M. *The Votive Statues of the Athenian Acropolis.* Cambridge: Cambridge University Press, 2003.

Keller, C. "Hatshepsut's Reputation in History." In *Hatshepsut from Queen to Pharaoh*, edited by C. A. Roehrig, 294–97. New York: Yale University Press, 2005.

Keller, C. "The Statuary of Hatshepsut." In *Hatshepsut from Queen to Pharaoh*, edited by C. A. Roehrig, 158–72. New York: Yale University Press, 2005.

Kemp, B. J. *Ancient Egypt: Anatomy of a Civilization.* London: Routledge, 1989.

Koch, N. J. *Picturae Initiis: Die Anfange der Griechischen Malerei im 7. Jahrhundert v.Chr.* Munich: Biering & Brinkmann, 1996.

Koch-Brinkmann, U. *Polychrome Bilder auf Weisgrundigen Lekythen.* Munich: Biering & Brinkmann, 1999.

Koloski-Ostrow, A. O., ed. *Naked Truths: Women, Sexuality and Gender in Classical Art.* London: Routledge, 1997.

Kozloff, A. P. *Amenhotep III: Egypt's Radiant Pharaoh*. New York: Cambridge University Press, 2011.

Kozloff, A. P. "Sculpture: An Overview." In *The Oxford Encyclopedia of Ancient Egypt*, Vol. 3, edited by D. B. Redford, 218–28. Oxford: Oxford University Press, 2001.

Kozloff, A. P., and B. M. Bryan. *Egypt's Dazzling Sun: Amenhotep III and His World*. Cleveland: Cleveland Museum of Art, 1992.

Kraus, R. "Akhetaten, a Portrait in Art of an Ancient Egyptian Capitol." In *Civilizations of the Ancient Near East*, edited by J. M. Sasson, 749. New York: Hendrickson Publishers, 1995.

Kreillinger, U. "To Be or Not to Be a Hetaira: Female Nudity in Classical Athens." In *Images and Gender: Contributions to the Hermeneutics of Reading Art*, edited by S. Schroer, 229–37. Fribourg: Vandenhoeck & Ruprecht, 2006.

Lacovara, P. "The City of Amarna." In *Pharaohs of the Sun*, edited by R. Freed, Y. Markowitz, and S. D'Auria, 61–71. Boston: Bulfinch Press, 1999.

Lang, F. "Structural Change in Archaic Greek Housing." In *Ancient Greek Houses and Households*, edited by B. Ault and L. Nevett, 12–35. Philadelphia: University of Pennsylvania Press, 2005.

Langdon, S. *Art and Identity in Dark Age Greece, 1100–700 BCE*. Cambridge: Cambridge University Press, 2008.

Lapatin, K. "Kerch Style Vases." In *The Colors of Clay: Special Techniques in Athenian Vases*, edited by B. Cohen, 317–41. Los Angeles: Getty Museum, 2006.

Lee, M. "Constructing Gender in the Feminine Greek Peplos." In *The Clothed Body in the Ancient World*, edited by L. Cleland, M. Harlow, and L. Llewellyn-Jones, 55–64. Oxford: Oxbow Books, 2005.

Lerner, G. *The Creation of Patriarchy*. Oxford: Oxford University Press, 1986.

Lesko, B. S. *The Great Goddesses of Egypt*. Norman: University of Oklahoma Press, 1991.

Lewis, S. *The Athenian Woman: An Iconographic Handbook*. London: Routledge, 2002.

Lissarrague, F. "Identity and Otherness: The Case of Attic Head Vases and Plastic Vases." *Source* 15, No. 1 (1995): 4–9.

Loden, T., ed. *The Language of Color in the Mediterranean*. Stockholm: Almquist & Wiksell International, 1999.

Lustig, J. "Kinship, Gender and Age in Middle Kingdom Tomb Scenes and Texts." In *Anthropology and Egyptology: A Developing Dialogue*, edited by J. Lustig, 43–66. London: Sheffield, 1997.

Lydakis, S. *Ancient Greek Painting and Its Echoes in Later Art*. Los Angeles: Getty Publications, 2002.

Lynch, K. M. "Erotic Images on Attic Vases: Markets and Meanings." In *Markets and Meanings: Athenian Potters and Painters*, edited by J. Oakley and O. Palagia, 159–65. Oxford: Oxford University Press, 2009.

Lyons, J. "The Vocabulary of Color with Particular Reference to Ancient Greek and Classical Latin." In *The Language of Color in the Mediterranean*, edited by T. Loden, 39–75. Stockholm: Almquist & Wiksell International, 1999.

Madrigal, L., and J. Kelly. "Human Skin-Color Sexual Dimorphism: A Test of the Sexual Selection Hypothesis." *American Journal of Physical Anthropology* 132 (2007): 470–82.

Malek, J. *Egypt: 4000 Years of Art*. London: Phaidon Press, 2003.

Mallinson, M. "The Sacred Landscape." In *Pharaohs of the Sun*, edited by R. Freed, Y. J. Markowitz, and E. D'Auria, 72–79. Boston: Bulfinch Press, 1999.

Manniche, L. "Sexuality." In *The Oxford Encyclopedia of Ancient Egypt*, edited by D. B. Redford, 274–76. Oxford: Oxford University Press, 2000.

Manzelli, V. "La Policromia Nella Statuaria Greca Arcaica." *Studia Archeologica* 69 (1994): 126–28. Rome.

Marinatos, N. *Art and Religion in Thera: Reconstructing a Bronze Age Society*. Athens: D & I Mathioulakis, 1984.

Marinatos, N. "The Bull as Adversary: Some Observations on Bull-hunting, Bull-leaping." In *Ariadne: Festschrift S. Alexiou*, 23–32. Herakleion: Rethymnon, 1989.

Martin, R., and F. Villard. *Archaic Greek Art, 620–480 BC*. London: Thames and Hudson, 1971.

Mattusch, C. *Greek Bronze Statuary from the Beginnings through the Fifth Century B.C.* Ithaca: Cornell University Press, 1988.

Mayo, M. E. *The Art of South Italy: Vases from Magna Graecia*. Richmond: Virginia Museum of Fine Arts, 1982.

McGlew, J. *Tyranny and Political Culture in Ancient Greece*. Ithaca: Cornell University Press, 1993.

McNiven, T. J. "Behaving Like an Other: Telltale Gestures in Athenian Vase Painting." In *Not the Classical Ideal: Athens and the Construction of the Other in Greek Art*, edited by B. Cohen, 71–97. Leiden: Brill Academic Publishers, 2000.

Mekhitarian, A. *Egyptian Painting*. New York: Rizzoli, 1978.

Meltzer, E. S. "Who Knows the Color of God?" *Journal of Ancient Civilizations* 11 (1996): 123–29.

Mertens, J. R. *Attic White-Ground: Its Development on Shapes Other than Lekythoi*. New York: Garland, 1977.

Mertens, J. R. "The Amasis Painter: Artist and Tradition." In *Papers on the Amasis Painter and His World*, 168–83. Malibu: Getty Museum, 1997.

Mertens, J. R. "Attic White Ground: Potter and Painter." In *The Colors of Clay: Special Techniques in Athenian Vases*, edited by B. Cohen, 186–94. Los Angeles: Getty Museum, 2006.

Mertens, J. R. *How to Read Greek Vases*. New York: Metropolitan Museum of Art, 2010.

Midant-Reyes, B. *The Pre-history of Egypt*. Translation by I. Shaw of 1997 original. Oxford: Wiley Blackwell, 2000.

Miller, M. C. "Myth of Bousiris." In *Not the Classical Ideal: Athens and the Construction of the Other in Greek Art*, edited by B. Cohen, 413–42. Leiden: Brill Academic Publishers, 2000.

Moortgat, A. *The Art of Ancient Mesopotamia*. London: Phaidon, 1969.

Morris, I. "Archaeology and Gender Ideologies in Early Archaic Greece." *Transactions of the American Philological Association* 129 (1999): 305–17.

Morris, I. *Archaeology as Cultural History: Words and Things in Iron Age Greece*. Malden, MA: Wiley-Blackwell, 2000.

Morris, S. P. *Daidalos and the Origins of Greek Art*. Princeton: Princeton University Press, 1992.

Morris, S. P. *The Black and White Style: Athens and Aegina in the Orientalizing Period*. New Haven: Yale University Press, 1994.

Morris, S. P. "Greek and Near Eastern Art in the Age of Homer." In *New Light on a Dark Age: Exploring the Culture of Geometric Greece*, edited by S. Langdon, 56–71. Columbia: University of Missouri Press, 1997.

Naerebout, F. G. "Male-Female Relationships in the Homeric Epics." In *Sexual Asymmetry: Studies in Ancient Society*, edited by J. Blok and P. Mason, 109–46. Amsterdam: J. C. Gieben, 1987.

Naville, E. *The Temple of Deir el-Bahri*, Part 2. London: Egypt Exploration Fund, 1896.

Neer, R. T. *Style and Politics in Athenian Vase-Painting: The Craft of Democracy, ca. 530–460 B. C. E.* Cambridge: Cambridge University Press, 2002.

Neer, R. T. *Greek Art and Archaeology: A New History, c. 2500–150 BCE*. New York: Thames and Hudson, 2012.

Neils, J. "Others Within the Other: An Intimate Look at Hetairai and Maeanads." In *Not the Classical Ideal: Athens and the Construction of the Other in Greek Art*, edited by B. Cohen, 203–26. Leiden: Brill Academic Publishers, 2000.

Neils, J. "Women Are White: White Ground and the Attic Funeral." In *Papers on Special Techniques in Athenian Vases*, edited by K. Lapatin, 61–70. Los Angeles: Getty Museum, 2008.

Nelson, S. *Gender in Archaeology: Analyzing Power and Prestige*. Walnut Creek, CA: AltaMira Press, 1999.

Nevett, L. *House and Society in the Ancient Greek World*. Cambridge: Cambridge University Press, 1999.

Nielsen, H. S. "Women in Classical Athens—Their Social Space: Ideal and Reality." In *Sex and Difference in Ancient Greece and Rome*, edited by M. G. Toohey, 23–30. Edinburgh: Edinburgh University Press, 2003.

Noble, V. *The Technique of Painted Attic Pottery*. Revised edition. London: Thames and Hudson, 1978.

Oakley, J. H. *Picturing Death in Classical Athens: The Evidence of the White Lekythoi*. New York: Cambridge University Press, 2004.

Oakley, J., and O. Palagia, eds. *Markets and Meanings: Athenian Potters and Painters*. Oxford: Oxford University Press, 2009.

Osborne, R. *Archaic and Classical Greek Art*. Oxford: Oxford University Press, 1998.

Padgett, J. M., ed. *The Centaur's Smile: The Human Animal in Early Greek Art*. New Haven: Yale University Press, 2003.

Papapostolou, J. A. "Colour in Ancient Painting." In *Color in Ancient Greece: The Role of*

Color in Ancient Greek Art and Architecture, 700–31 BC, edited by M. A. Tiverios and D. S. Tsiafakis, 53–64. Thessaloniki, 2002.

Parrot, A. *Sumer.* London: Golden Press, 1960.

Parrot, A. *Ninevah and Babylon.* London: Thames and Hudson, 1961.

Payne, H. *Necrocorinthia: A Study of Corinthian Art in the Archaic Period.* Oxford: Clarendon Press, 1931.

Pedley, J. G. *Greek Art and Archaeology.* Upper Saddle River, NJ: Prentice-Hall, 2007.

Phillips, K. M., Jr. "Perseus and Andromeda." *American Journal of Archaeology* 72 (1968): 1–23.

Pinney, G. *Figures of Speech, Men and Maidens in Ancient Greece.* Chicago: University of Chicago Press, 2002.

Platnauer, M. "Greek Colour-Perception." *Classical Quarterly*, 15, Nos. 3 and 4 (1921): 153–62.

Plumley, J. M. "Qasr Ibrîm." *Journal of Egyptian Archaeology* 61 (1975): 212–38.

Pollitt, J. J. *The Art of Ancient Greece: Sources and Documents.* Cambridge: Cambridge University Press, 1993.

Pollock, S. *Ancient Mesopotamia: The Eden that Never Was.* Cambridge: Cambridge University Press, 1999.

Pollock, S., and R. Bernbeck. "And They Said, Let Us Make Gods in Our Image: Gendered Ideologies in Ancient Mesopotamia." In *Reading the Body: Representations and Remains in the Archaeological Record*, edited by A. Rautman, 150–64. Philadelphia: University of Pennsylvania Press, 2000.

Pomeroy, S. *Goddesses, Whores, Wives and Slaves: Women in Classical Antiquity.* New York: Schocken, 1975.

Popham, M. "An Engraved Near Eastern Bronze Bowl from Lefkandi." *Oxford Journal of Archaeology*, 14 (1995), 103–7.

Preziosi, D., and L. A. Hitchcock. *Aegean Art and Architecture.* Oxford: Oxford University Press, 1999.

Rasmussen, T. "Corinth and Orientalizing." In *Looking at Greek Vases*, edited by T. Rasmussen and N. Spivey, 57–78. Cambridge: Cambridge University Press, 1991.

Rautman, A., ed. *Reading the Body: Representations and Remains in the Archaeological Record.* Philadelphia: University of Pennsylvania Press, 2000.

Redford, D. B. *History and Chronology of the Eighteenth Dynasty of Egypt: Seven Studies.* Toronto: University of Toronto Press, 1967.

Redford, D. B. "East Karnak and the Sed-Festival of Akhenaten." In *Hommages à Jean Leclant I: Études pharaoniques*, 485–87. Cairo, 1994.

Redford, D. B. "The Beginning of the Heresy." In *Pharaohs of the Sun*, edited by R. Freed, Y. Markowitz, and S. D'Auria, 50–61. Boston: Bulfinch Press, 1999.

Redford, D. B., ed. *The Oxford Encyclopedia of Ancient Egypt.* Oxford: Oxford University Press, 2001.

Reeder, E. D. "Representing Women." In *Pandora: Women in Classical Greece*, edited by E. D. Reeder, 123–94. Princeton: Princeton University Press, 1995.

Reusser, C. *Vasen für Etrurien: Verbreitung und Funktionen attische Keramik im Etrurien des 6.und 5. Jahrhunderts vor Christus*. Zurich: Akanthus, 2002.

Rice, M. *Egypt's Making: The Origins of Ancient Egypt (5000–2000 B.C)*. London: Routledge, 2003.

Ridgway, B. S. *The Archaic Style in Greek Sculpture*. Chicago: Ares Publications, 1993.

Ridgway, B. S. *Prayers in Stone: Greek Architectural Sculpture*. Berkeley: University of California Press, 1999.

Robertson, M. *A History of Greek Art*. Cambridge: Cambridge University Press, 1975.

Robertson, M. *The Art of Vase-Painting in Classical Athens*. Cambridge: Cambridge University Press, 1992.

Robins, G. *Women in Ancient Egypt*. Cambridge: Harvard University Press, 1993.

Robins, G. "Some Principles of Compositional Dominance and Gender Hierarchy in Egyptian Art." *Journal of the American Research Center in Egypt*, 31 (1994): 33–40.

Robins, G. *Proportion and Style in Ancient Egyptian Art*. Austin: University of Texas Press, 1994.

Robins, G. *Reflections of Women in the New Kingdom: Ancient Egyptian Art from the New Kingdom*. Atlanta: Emory University, 1995.

Robins, G. "Dress, Undress and the Representation of Fertility and Potency in New Kingdom Egyptian Art." In *Sexuality in Ancient Art*, edited by N. B. Kampen, 27–40. Cambridge: Cambridge University Press, 1996.

Robins, G. *The Art of Ancient Egypt*. Cambridge: Cambridge University Press, 1997.

Robins, G. "The Names of Hatshepsut as King." *Journal of Egyptian Archaeology* 85 (1999): 109–12.

Robins, G. "Gender Roles." In *The Oxford Encyclopedia of Ancient Egypt*, Vol. 2, edited by D. B. Redford, 12–16. Oxford: Oxford University Press, 2000.

Robins, G. "Color Symbolism." In *The Oxford Encyclopedia of Ancient Egypt*, Vol. 1, edited by D. B. Redford, 291–94. Oxford: Oxford University Press, 2001.

Robins, G. "Women." In *The Oxford Encyclopedia of Ancient Egypt*,Vol. 3, edited by D. B. Redford, 510–16. Oxford: Oxford University Press, 2001.

Rocco, G. *La ceramagrafia protoattica: pittori e botteghe (710–630 a.c.)*. Rahden/Westff: VML, Verlag Marie Leidorf, 2008.

Roehrig, C. H. "Women's Work: Some Occupations of Nonroyal Women as Depicted in Ancient Egyptian Art." In *Mistress of the House, Mistress of Heaven: Women in Ancient Egypt*, edited by A. Capel and G. Markoe, 19–24. New York: Cincinnati Art Museum, 1996.

Roehrig, C. H., ed. *Hatshepsut from Queen to Pharaoh*. New York: Metropolitan Museum of Art, 2005.

Roth, A. M. "Father Earth, Mother Sky: Ancient Egyptian Beliefs about Conception and

Fertility." In *Reading the Body: Representations and Remains in the Archaeological Record*, edited by A. Rautman, 187–201. Philadelphia: University of Pennsylvania Press, 2000.

Roth, A. M. "Models of Authority: Hatshepsut's Predecessors in Power." In *Hatshepsut from Queen to Pharaoh*, edited by C. H. Roehrig, 9–15. New York: Metropolitan Museum of Art, 2005.

Roth, A. M. "Erasing a Reign." In *Hatshepsut from Queen to Pharaoh*, edited by C. H. Roehrig, 277–83. New York: Metropolitan Museum of Art, 2005.

Rystedt, E., and B. Wells, eds. *Pictorial Pursuits: Figurative Painting on Mycenaen and Geometric Pottery, papers from two seminars at the Swedish Institute at Athens in 1999 and 2001*. Stockholm: Svenska Institutet, 2006.

Sandman, M. *Texts from the Time of Akhenaten*. Brussels: Fondation Egyptologique Reine, 1938.

Savage, S. "The Status of Women in Pre-Dynastic Egypt as Revealed through Mortuary Analysis." In *Reading the Body: Representations and Remains in the Archaeological Record*, edited by A. Rautmann, 77–92. Philadelphia: University of Pennsylvania Press, 2000.

Saxonhouse, A. W. *Fear of Diversity: The Birth of Political Science in Ancient Greek Thought*. Chicago: University of Chicago Press, 1992.

Schäfer, H. *Principles of Egyptian Art.*, Edited by Emma Brunner-Traut. Translated by John Baines. Oxford: Griffith Institute, 1974.

Schaus, G. P. "The Beginning of Greek Polychrome Painting." *Journal of Hellenic Studies* 108 (1988): 107–17.

Scheibler, I. "Features and Intentions of Color-Schemes in Archaic Vase-Painting." In *Color in Ancient Greece: The Role of Color in Ancient Greek Art and Architecture (700–31 BC)*, edited by M. A. Tiverios and D. S. Tsiafakis, 65–75. Thessaloniki, 2002.

Schroer, S., ed. *Images and Gender: Contributions to the Hermeneutics of Reading Art*. Fribourg: Vandenhoeck & Ruprecht, 2006.

Sellers, E. *The Elder Pliny's Chapters on the History of Art*. Translated by K. Jex-Blake. New York: Macmillan, 1896.

Shanks, M. *Art and the Early Greek State: An Interpretive Archaeology*. Cambridge: Cambridge University Press, 1999.

Shanks, M. "Art and Archaeology of Embodiment: Some Aspects of Archaic Greece." *Cambridge Archaeological Journal* 5, No. 2 (1999): 207–44.

Shapiro, H. A. "Autochthony and the Visual Arts." In *Democracy and the Arts in Fifth-Century Athens*, edited by D. Boedeker and K. A. Raaflaub. 127–51. Cambridge: Harvard University Press, 1998.

Shaw, M. C. "The Priest King Fresco from Knossos: Man, Woman, Priest, King or Someone Else?" In *ΧΑΡΙΣ: Essays in Honor of Sara A. Immerwahr*, Hesperia Supplement 33, edited by A. P. Chapin, 65–83. Athens, 2004.

Shefold, K. *Myth and Legend in Early Greek Art*. New York: Harry N. Abrams, 1966.

Silverblatt, I. "Women in States." *Annual Review of Anthropology* 17 (1988): 427–60.

Small, D. B. "An Archaeology of Democracy." In *Archaeological Institute of America Colloquia and Conference Papers, No. 2: Democracy 2500? Questions and Challenges*, edited by I. Morris and K. A. Raaflaub, 217–18. Dubuque: Kendall/Hunt Publishing, 1997.

Smith , C. A. "Proto-Attic Vase." *Journal of Hellenic Studies* 22 (1902): 29–45.

Smith, S. T. "Race." In *The Oxford Encyclopedia of Ancient Egypt*, Vol. 3, edited by D. B. Redford, 111–16. Oxford: Oxford University Press, 2001.

Smith, W. S. *The Art and Architecture of Ancient Egypt*. Revised by W. K. Simpson. New Haven: Yale University Press, 1981. First published 1958.

Smith, W. S. *Ancient Egypt as Represented in the Museum of Fine Arts, Boston*. Boston: T. O. Metcalf, 1960.

Snodgrass, A. *Archaic Greece: The Age of Experiment*. London: J. M. Dent and Sons, 1980.

Snowden, F. *Blacks in Antiquity*. Cambridge: Belknap Press, 1970.

Snowden, F. *Before Color Prejudice: The Ancient View of Blacks*. Cambridge: Harvard University Press, 1983.

Snowden, F. "Greeks and Ethiopians." In *Greeks and Barbarians: Essays on the Interactions between Greeks and Non-Greeks and the Consequences for Eurocentrism*, edited by J. Coleman and C. A. Walz, 103–6. Bethesda, MD: Capital Decisions, 1997.

Spanel, D. *Through Ancient Eyes: Egyptian Portraiture*. Birmingham, AL: University of Washington Press, 1988.

Spycket, A. *La Statuaire du Proche-Orient ancien*. Cologne: Brill Academic Publishers, 1981.

Stansbury-O'Donnell, M. D. *Vase Painting, Gender and Social Identity in Archaic Athens*. Cambridge: Cambridge University Press, 2006.

Steel, L. "Women in Mycenaean Pictorial Vase Painting." In *Pictorial Pursuits: Figurative Painting on Mycenaean and Geometric Pottery, papers from two seminars at the Swedish Institute at Athens in 1999 and 2001*, edited by E. Rystedt and B. Wells, 147–55. Stockholm: Svenska Institutet, 2006.

Stewart, A. "Imag(in)ing the Other: Amazons and Ethnicity in Fifth-Century Athens." *Poetics Today* 16 (1995): 571–97.

Stewart, A. *Art, Desire and the Body in Ancient Greece*. Cambridge: Cambridge University Press, 1997.

Stewart, A. *Classical Greece and the Birth of Western Art*. Cambridge: Cambridge University Press, 2008.

Strauss, B. S. "Ideology and Society in Democratic Athens." In *Archaeological Institute of America Colloquia and Conference Papers*, No. 2: *Democracy 2500? Questions and Challenges*, edited by I. Morris and K. A. Raaflaub, 141–54. Dubuque: Kendall/Hunt Publishing, 1997.

Sutton, R. F., Jr. *The Interaction between Men and Women Portrayed on Attic Red-Figure Pottery*. Chapel Hill: University of North Carolina, 1981.

Sutton, R. F. "The Good, the Base and the Ugly: The Drunken Orgy in Attic Vase Painting and the Athenian Self." In *Not the Classical Ideal: Athens and the Construction of the Other in Greek Art*, edited by B. Cohen, 180–202. Leiden: Brill Academic Publishers, 2000.

Sutton, R. F. "Family Portraits: Recognizing the Oikos on Attic Red Figure Pottery." In *ΧΑΡΙΣ: Essays in Honor of Sara A. Immerwahr*, Hesperia Supplement 33, edited by A. Chapin, 327–50.Princeton: American School of Classical Studies, 2004.

Swindler, M. H. *Ancient Painting*. New Haven: AMS Press, 1929.

Teeter, E. *Ancient Egypt: Treasures from the Collection of the Oriental Institute*. Chicago: University of Chicago, 1999.

Tefnin, R. *La statuaire d' Hatshepsout: Portrait royal et politique sous la 18e Dynastie*. Brussels: Fondation Egyptologique Reine, 1997.

Tefnin, R. "Sculpture: Private Sculpture." In *The Oxford Encyclopedia of Ancient Egypt*, Vol. 3, edited by D. B. Redford, 218–28. Oxford: Oxford University Press, 2001.

Tiverios, M. A., and D. S. Tsiafakis, eds. *Color in Ancient Greece*. Thessaloniki, 2002.

Tobin, V. A. "Creation Myths." In *The Oxford Encyclopedia of Ancient Egypt*, Vol. 1, edited by D. B. Redford, 469–72. Oxford: Oxford University Press, 2001.

Trigger, B. "Egyptology, Ancient Egypt and the American Imagination." In *The American Discovery of Ancient Egypt*, edited by N. Thomas, 21–35. Los Angeles: Los Angeles County Museum, 1995.

Troy, L. *Patterns of Queenship in Ancient Egyptian Myth and History*. Upsala: Acta Universitatis Upsaliensis, 1986.

True, M. "Plastic Vases and Vases with Plastic Additions: Athenian Potters and the Production of Plastic Vases." In *The Colors of Clay: Special Techniques in Athenian Vases*, edited by B. Cohen, 239–90. Los Angeles: Getty Museum, 2006.

Tsiafakis, D. "ΠΕΛΩΡΑ: Fabulous Creatures and/or Demons of Death?" In *The Centaur's Smile: The Human Animal in Early Greek Art*, 73–104. New Haven: Yale University Press, 2003.

Tydesley, J. *Daughters of Isis*. London: Penguin, 1994.

Tydesley, J. *Hatchepsut*. London: Penguin, 1996.

Tydesley, J. *Chronicles of the Queens of Egypt*. London: Thames and Hudson, 2006.

Vermeule, E. D. T. "Painted Mycenaean Larnakes." *Journal of Hellenic Studies* 85 (1965): 123–48.

Vermeule, E., and V. Karageorghis. *Mycenaean Pictorial Vase-Painting*. Cambridge: Harvard University Press, 1982.

Vinson, S. "Narmer." In *The Oxford Encyclopedia of Ancient Egypt*, Vol. 2, edited by D. B. Redford, 494–95. Oxford: Oxford University Press, 2001.

Viswerseram, K. "Race and the Culture of Anthropology." *American Anthropologist* 100 (1998): 70–83.

von Bothmer, D. *The Amasis Painter and His World*. New York: Thames and Hudson, 1985.

Walter-Karydi, E. "Prinzipien der archaischen Farbgebung." In *Studien Zur Klassischen Archäologie, Festschrift für Friedrich Hiller*, edited by F. Hiller and K. Braun, 23–41. Saarbrücken, 1986.

Watrous, L. V. "The Origin and Iconography of the Late Minoan Painted Larnax." *Hesperia*, 60, No. 3 (1991): 285–307.

Weatherhead, F. "Recording and Conservation of Painted Plaster from the Early Excavations at Amarna." In *Colour and Painting in Ancient Egypt*, edited by W. V. Davies, 53–59. London: British Museum Press, 2000.

Webster's New Universal Unabridged Dictionary. New York: Barnes and Noble, 1996.

Wehgartner, I. *Attische weisgrunde Keramik. Maltechniken, Werkstätten, Formen, Verwendung*. Mainz: Von Zabern, 1983.

Westenholz, J. G. "Goddesses of the Ancient Near East, 3000–1000 BC." In *Ancient Goddesses*, edited by L. Goodison and C. Morris, 63–82. Madison: University of Wisconsin, 1998.

Whitley, J. "Proto-Attic Pottery: A Contextual Approach." In *Classical Greece: Ancient Histories and Modern Archaeologies*, edited by I. Morris, 57–70. Cambridge: Cambridge University Press, 1994.

Wilkinson, C. K., and M. Hill. *Egyptian Wall Paintings*. New York: Abbeville Press, 1983.

Wilkinson, R. H. *Reading Egyptian Art*. London: Thames and Hudson, 1982.

Wilkinson, R. H. *Symbol and Magic in Egyptian Art*. London: Thames and Hudson, 1994.

Wilkinson, T. A. H. *Early Dynastic Egypt*. New York: Routledge, 1999.

Winter, I. "Women in Public: The Disk of Enheduanna, the Beginning of the Office of EN-Priestess and the Weight of Visual Evidence." In *La Femme dans le Proche-Orient Antique*, edited by J. M. Durand, 189–201. Paris: Rencontre Assyriologique Internationale, 1987.

Zanker, P. *The Power of Images in the Age of Augustus*. Ann Arbor: University of Michigan Press, 1988.

Zeitlin, F. *Playing the Other: Gender and Society in Classical Greek Literature*. Chicago: University of Chicago Press, 1996.

Index

Page locators in *italics* indicate photographs.